BODYBUILDING

Everything You Need to Know About Bodybuilding

(How to Quantify Your Bodybuilding and
Transform Your Physiqu)

Bryan Mackey

Published By Andrew Zen

Bryan Mackey

All Rights Reserved

Bodybuilding: Everything You Need to Know About Bodybuilding (How to Quantify Your Bodybuilding and Transform Your Physiqu)

ISBN 978-1-77485-282-8

Legal & Disclaimer

The information contained in this book is not designed to replace or take the place of any form of medicine or professional medical advice. The information in this book has been provided for educational and entertainment purposes only.

The information contained in this book has been compiled from sources deemed reliable, and it is accurate to the best of the Author's knowledge; however, the Author cannot guarantee its accuracy and validity and cannot be held liable for any errors or omissions. Changes are periodically made to this book. You must consult your doctor or get professional medical advice before using any of the suggested remedies, techniques, or information in this book.

Upon using the information contained in this book, you agree to hold harmless the Author from and against any damages, costs, and expenses, including any legal fees potentially resulting from the application of any of the information provided by this guide. This disclaimer applies to any damages or injury caused by the use and application, whether directly or indirectly, of any advice or information presented, whether for breach of contract, tort, negligence, personal injury, criminal intent, or under any other cause of action.

You agree to accept all risks of using the information presented inside this book. You need to consult a professional medical practitioner in order to ensure you are both able and healthy enough to participate in this program.

TABLE OF CONTENTS

Introduction

It's been my experience in the fitness business for 33 years as a gym's owner personal trainer, and bodybuilding coach. In that time I've observed some fascinating aspects of the bodies of women. The '80s were when Jazzercise was a huge trend. The 1990s saw the emergence of Tae-bo. In the '00's, there was Cross-Fit as women gradually began to realize the benefits of training with weights.

Over the last three decades, I've assisted hundreds of women change their body from sluggish to fab and transformed them in bodybuilding champions. Utilizing bodybuilding techniques that have helped these women move away from the misconceptions surrounding women and weights , causing massive physical transformations all over their bodies. The book I'll expose the same methods in diet, training and nutrition that have led to these tough bodies. If you follow this guide, you can transform your body and training.

The decision to pursue a bodybuilding routine will create a stronger and fitter person. It will also develop inside you the essential qualities that will allow you achieve success throughout your life . . .

Discipline

Confidence

Perseverance

Okay, are you ready to take that first step?

It's time to put the finishing touches on your soft self and begin to harden to the max...

Chapter 1: Building Muscle and Burning Fat

Individuals who are looking to work out are often asking Is it possible to increase strength and muscle mass without adding the fat? Recent studies have proven that it's possible however, it isn't easy.

A study provided significant new evidence for this seemingly impossible goal. The study involved 40 teens who endured the gruelling exercise for four weeks and at the same time decreasing the amount of amount of energy they had available by 40. These men were not in top shape, and they wanted to shed some of their weight , while conserving their muscle mass and increasing their endurance. All participants were fed an calorie-controlled diet and then split into 2 groups. One group was given a greater amount of protein than the other. When the study the high protein group had significant increases in muscle mass and other groups had little or no gain in muscle; however they didn't lose any muscles. The group with high protein also shed more weight than the other groups.

What happened in the end? To better understand what happened we need to look at the biology that underlies the process. We know that the body is able to break down muscles when we eat but what exactly is the reason? When we decrease the calories consumed and energy, we lose it proportionally. In some way, our bodies must make up for the loss. In order to do this it makes use of the fats that we carry together with the proteins we have in our muscles to produce sugars in order to generate energy. This means that if there's enough proteins in blood and the body is not need to pull it from muscles. The best way to make sure of this is to consume lots of protein! When you say "plenty," strive to attain 1-1/2 grams of protein for every kilogram of body weight each day.

Another important thing to consider is homeostasis. The term "homeostasis" refers to the specific nature of the body to remain at the place it is. The body is not able to tolerate changes like losing or gaining weight , and is equipped with its very own system that is designed to stop the incoming changes. In this way, it ensures constant levels of temperature as well as other factors like salt, sugar proteins, fats, calcium , and oxygen levels within the blood.Similar systems constantly maintain stable state of the earth's ecosystem.

The human body employs many various processes to manage its temperature and maintain a average that is 98.6 F. If the body gets too hot, sweating can occur which makes the skin likely to evaporate. Balance is also at work. If an athlete sweats excessively, it is an indication to reduce their pace and cool down.

It is evident that the condition the body's in can be of vital significance. At any time your body can be in either an anabolic, or catabolic state.

"Anabolic" refers to a term used to describe a situation in which complex structures are constructed by combining simpler elements. "Catabolic" is the exact opposite, simplifying complex structures into simpler ones. This means that, with a handful of variations, it's extremely difficult for the majority of people to build muscle without eating a lot of fat.

The subject we're talking about is your metabolism, an array of systems in your body which allow for the exchange of matter and energy with the outside world.

As humans, we depend on our metabolism to function and grow daily. Certain biological (without existence) systems are created externally, such as iron rust. The metabolism of our body is the process that allows us to keep our structure and our well-organized molecules in a stable state. Our metabolism is comprised of two kinds of dependent phases: one in which energy is used and the other in which energy is absorbed.

Catabolism is a process where complex organic compounds break down to release energy. Anabolism is the process when the complex organic molecules are made from simpler substances to store energy. Catabolism is when cells absorb molecules, like glucose from their surroundings and break it down and release the energy. When the energy is released, it is absorbed by the specially-designed molecules ATP. If the energy accumulated by an action by ATP is used to make new compounds that are more complicated, this process is known as anabolism.

In general, the substances soaked from the catabolic phase will be utilized in the anabolic phase.

Carbohydrates are the primary energy source for us. Second are lipids, which we turn in the event that carbs become exhausted, or in their own way when needed. The most powerful organic compounds is found in proteins -- the first option when it comes to creating structures or regulating processes.

Whole Grains: the first choice for obtaining carbohydrates for your diet ought to be whole grain. High in minerals, vitamins antioxidants as well as healthy fats and fiber Whole grains are brimming with nutrients found in nature. substituting whole grains in place of refined grains such as white bread that are often present in our diets may reduce the risk of developing heart disease and diabetes. Whole grain food items include wild rice and quinoa, as well as whole wheat breads, popcorn, and whole wheat pasta.

The more vibrant your fruit basket is, the better. Fruits are not high in fat, calories and salt as well as calories. They are also loaded with vital nutrients that we typically do not consume, such as potassium, which could aid in reducing blood pressure as well as vitamin C and the folic acid. Fruits are a great source of disease fighting agents and help in lowering blood cholesterol, and could reduce the risk of developing heart disease. Fiber is essential for maintaining good bowel function. Fruits help you feel fuller and has fewer calories.

Pick up blackberries, prunes dried peaches and apricots melons, orange juice, bananas, blueberries, pears Apples, cherries, and pineapple. Be sure to incorporate fruits into your diet. Eat 4-5 servings a day.

Beans: let's cheer for beans. They are so high in nutrients that they're thought of as both a vegetable and a protean. Beans are an excellent source of zinc, iron folate, iron, and of obviously, protein.Help manage your blood sugar levels by adding lots of beans into your diet. Beans may also lower cholesterol levels and triglyceride levels. They can even lower blood pressure.Beans are often referred to as the superfood. They are generally between 2 and 3 percent fat and have no cholesterol , unless coupled with other ingredients, for example, Lard. They may also help to keep your blood sugar level stable because of their complex carbohydrates. They can also help to reduce irritability and fatigue.

Enjoy them as salads or soup, as well as rice dishes.

Vegetables: your diet must consist of plenty of low-calorie, nutrient-rich and high-quality carbohydrates that are found in vegetables. They naturally are low in calories and fats as well as containing vitamins C and A along with folate and potassium as well as fiber. Studies have proven that these essential foods can reduce the risk of heart disease as well as certain cancers, type 2 diabetes, and weight gain. Plants that are rich in potassium include sweet and white potatoes beet greens, white beans tomatoes, tomato sauce and juice as well as lima beans, spinach, as well as kidney beans.

Milk: you might be shocked to learn that milk is a great source of carbohydrates, with 1/2 cup of it containing the same amount as one slice of whole-wheat bread.Milk is a good carb because of its bone-friendly amount of calcium and vitamin D as well as protein. A low-fat or fat-free diet is the most suitable option.

If anabolic processes prevail within a cell, then growth will continue. If cells have developed fully, between two states, a healthy equilibrium will be maintained. This is particularly true in children, where growth that is healthy is the goal. Children's natural ability to heal quickly and recover from illness has been observed. However, as adults, we need to maintain the balance between these two tasks to sustain our bodies.

As we get older, our balance can gradually shift towards the catabolic end of the spectrum, bringing upon the changes in our energy that which we imagine when we think of "elder." As we age, our bodies gradually lose the ability to keep pace with the process of breakdown that is happening inside us. We feel a decrease in energy, the deterioration of our physical functions and a higher chance of suffering from injuries and illnesses. We are more prone to fall and suffer ailments and infections that last for a long time. A key factor in battling this depressing condition is living a healthy life, that includes regular exercise, plenty of rest, and a balanced diet.

Another option to prevent this is to supplement with supplements and botanicals that aid in anabolic activity. You should look for amino acids present in diet and supplements, magnesium, high-quality herbal extracts; and superfoods such as Whey protein, all of which contribute to anabolic metabolism.

"Bulking" refers to the act of putting onto weight (including fat) which is usually followed by a frantic effort to lose weight which is known as "cutting." The term "bulk" and cutting as a technique is frequently used by people looking to chisel their muscles. Many of us have discovered by experience that weight can be awe-inspiringly quick to gain, but painfully slow to remove. Thirty pounds gained in the course of a month could take years to shed and it's certainly not the same as the process of putting it on!

If you're absolutely eager to build muscles without adding weight This is how you can achieve it.

The first thing to remember is that fat is a major source of fat when we consume more calories than we require to keep our body weight in check. You should aim for an adequate amount of calories. A ratio of 16 times the weight of your body in pounds is the best. For instance, if you have 175 pounds, and aiming to gainweight, aim to consume 2800 calories per day. Every calorie should be filled with nutrients and vitamins in order to build muscle mass and speed up the recovery time. The empty calories are exactly that empty. Foods with no calories include snacks, chips, packaged foods and soda. They could contain sugar.

If you are looking to build muscle mass while also preventing weight gain, you must pay attention to what you put into your body. Choose healthy foods: fats, lean protein , and healthy carbs that are full of nutrients.

You've probably heard that muscles are comprised of proteins. This is almost accurate. Protein is comprised of amino acids that are vital to build an energised body and for healing the damage. Much more important than the amount of protein you consume is the type of protein you consume. Choose high-quality source of protein, and you'll be already on your way to building muscle mass without dramatically increasing the amount of fat in your body. Quality protein can be found in lean ground meat egg whites, chicken breasts of chicken and fish, and other high quality protein supplements.

Another benefit of protein is that although carbs boost insulin levels in your body, protein doesn't matter for those who are diabetic. The higher the insulin level, the more fat you'll keep. Be sure to get enough protein and eliminate carbs.

However, that doesn't mean carbs are not important. They are vital and are also healthy fats. Remember to think about the quality. It is also important to know the amount of carbs your body is able to convert into it, and then use them wisely instead of depending on cravings or occasions such as the dinner you have at Aunt Mary's. If your carbs are out of hand, your insulin level will increase and you'll gain weight. Good carbs give your muscles energy. In contrast, bad carbs make you exhausted. The best carbs are those that are fiber-rich, nutritious foods like sugary potatoes, brown rice oatmeal, and many more.

In the past, people used to believe that fats were bad for your health. Some people still do. If you're looking to gain weight, plenty of calories are found in fats, including 9 calories per grams. Carbs and proteins are next with 4 calories per gram. However, more calories could be bad and I'm not looking to be fat!

The difference lies on the caliber of calories you consume when you are aiming for a strong muscle mass and quality is the primary most important thing. Carbs and fats that are of high quality. Good fats include olive oil and olives, avocados, nuts and fish. These fats contain nutrients that can help enhance your eyesight and provide healthier hair, nails and skin. Fish oil included in the diet could provide the same advantages. There are studies that suggest that omega-3 fats that are found in fish, and in other foods can help cause fat to be burned as a consequence. These processed fats, like butter, potato chips as well as many salad dressings and margarine aren't have this effect, and are considered a "no-no."

This nutritional advice will not help you in the absence of working out frequently, so go to the gym or go out and run, lift weights, or race along using your rowing device. Find a workout routine that is suitable for your lifestyle as well as makes you feel comfortable and you'll have the chance to build muscle and staying clear of flab.

Another thing that doesn't help you is not working out regularly. It is essential to follow your workout routine every day or even every other day regardless of how you've created it. Set it as a priority, in addition to brushing your teeth, and eating a nutritious breakfast. There's no reason to work on building muscles and then losing it once you stop focusing. If you can make your exercise into a routine that you stick to, it will benefit you well. Keep in mind that the mind controls the body. If you set your mind to establish a routine of exercising the body might be reluctant to comply but it will follow through and do it without a lot of whining when you stick to your routine. It will eventually become used to your workout routine that it won't even complain if you don't.

Chapter 2: The Body, And Its Environment

The body can be affected by numerous factors, both external or internal. Chapter 2's title is about external influences but a brief discussion of aspects within the body wouldn't harm.

Internal aspects:

There are times when you will come across an individual in the gym, who is exercising with flu Don't do it! Avoid that! People who do this will just exhaust themselves, and can make others in their vicinity sick! If you are feeling sick or are about to become sick, allow your body its due rest to aid in strengthening your immune system.

Another aspect to consider is our psychological state that can be the reason we aren't achieving our goals, or even just the "mood" to avoid hitting the exercise. If we're not feeling fatigued or physically tired and mentally, we can find in our self some good ways of to bring out some feelings that can aid us.And we've already dealt with this at the beginning of this article.

External elements:

It is a fact that life is full of unpredictable events! This could constitute one of the elements that affect our exercise routine. So, how do we manage this issue?

The best method to handle unexpected situations is to be flexible! This implies having the capacity to alter our plans in response to the circumstances that come our ways.

Since the majority of us have a tight schedules and a lot of obligations to meet most of us tend to place working out in the middle of their tasks list.

What many people do not realize is that staying physical active is on our foremost priority list. A brief discussion of this is needed physical activity, it improves our mood, boost our energy levels, and boost our overall health. This enables us to cope better with our busy schedules and commitments.

One important thing to avoid is enrolling at a gym that is far from your work or home. As you can imagine, this could increase the chance of having you stop going to the fitness center.

Social assistance:

Social support from friends can keep you on track with those fitness targets. A fitness coach is an ideal idea! It might be an individual trainer, or an intimate friend who has already a fitness enthusiast.

Furthermore, a night out with a buddy is a good idea as well. It is possible to do this by exercising simultaneously at the fitness center. Thus, you'll be encouraging one another and will be able to give each other spots as required.

Posture:

Posture is just one of the numerous benefits we can enjoy by staying physically active and following an exercise routine that is effective. It's the posture where we keep our body in a straight line against gravity of standing, in a sitting position or lying down. Correct posture helps reduce stress and enhances the strength of every joints.

Many people are physically active, but have an unsteady posture! Poor posture can be the result of the work environment, bad habits, or even from everyday actions.

The first thing is that we need to be aware of what the ideal posture for different sittings.Being conscious of it every day, will assist us in improving it. For instance, if are spending a lot of time at the desk, take note of the way you hold yourself as well as if your lower and upper back are properly aligned.

How we walk may affect our posture as well. Many people walk with their front torso bent forward and curving their backs! The correct method is to stand up with your chest out and pressed with your head straight. bring your stomach back and lightly pull the core muscles tight "to ensure that our abdominal muscles help support our posture while walking" and walk with your hips. Strong abdominal muscles, as well as glutes, can help to support the upper body when walking.

The last but not least doing some stretching or yoga classes can help enhance our muscle balance around joints, and increase our joint range of motion which will eventually result in a better posture.

Being conscious of our bodies and our surroundings can be habit for some, and something that should be practiced for all of us. As we've said that we must be aware of our internal, external influences that can affect our wellbeing. Additionally, we should seek out or create an online community to support us when we need it. Also, we should be aware of posture a regular regularly until it becomes an automatic reflex.

Chapter 3: Diet For Weight Loss

While weight loss is the principal goal, it's essential to make sure you're maintaining your well-being. Remember to never overeat! If you stay true the CMV you have set, the goal to lose weight is achieved. The sources of these calories are crucial to be aware of too. The chapter details the food items and drinks you can but not consume.

Foods and Drinks to Be Refrain from

You must make a serious effort to avoid eating the food items listed in the below list. The consumption of these foods could result in a major or a slight reversal in your weight loss regimen based on the amount.

Fast food

Trans-fat-rich foods are high in trans-fats.

Soft drinks

Foods that have a significant amount of sodium and sugar.

Refraining from these foods will not only help in losing weight, but also keeps your body in good shape. The results of scientific research have shown that these food items and drinks could be dangerous to our body. They could lead to obesity, leading to heart problems and, therefore, should be kept away from.

Foods and Drinks that Can be consumed

As well as avoiding the previously mentioned foods, it's imperative to follow an "balanced eating plan". It is eating a balanced diet with optimal amounts of three elements from which people gain calories, carbohydrates, proteins, and fats. The practice of eating a diet that consume almost nothing is not the best approach to dieting. They're bound to result in the loss of weight, but they can have negative consequences for our bodies. So, nutritionists have developed the concept of a balanced diet that is consumed to ensure good health. It is important to combine this with exercising and avoiding the food items mentioned above to shed weight effectively.

Nutrients that are Essential For Balanced Diets

Protein

The USDA suggests a minimum of 0.8 grams of protein daily for each kilogram of body weight for an average adult. Since you'll be exercising to shed weight, the recommended amount of protein consumption is about a quarter the weight of your body per day. The calculation is different for those who weigh differently. Overweight people should consider their weight target in order to calculate their protein they consume, not their weight. Someone who is in the normal weight category could apply their weight at the moment.

Below are the sources of protein:

Dairy products, such as milk and cheese

Eggs

Meat

Fish and oils from fish

Fat

The USDA suggests that a minimum thirty percent (or 30%) of calories consumed must be from fats. This is the recommended amount for an average adult. Specialists from the field of nutrition have advised that the amount fats that the body needs to consume ranges from 20-30 percent.

When people hear the word fat, they tend to be scared of it. What they don't know is there's various kinds of fat, and some are essential to your body. There are four kinds of fats:

Transfat

Saturated Fat

Polyunsaturated fat

Monounsaturated fat

Of the four kinds of fats, the first two kinds of fat are the ones you must stay clear of if you're looking to lose weight. You may want to limit your consumption of saturated fats but you should also consider avoiding transfat completely. The kinds of foods you may prefer to stay clear of include fast food, chips and pastries, as well as snacks. It is essential to stay clear of junk food and junk food in any form.

The two kinds of fat are the ones you should consider taking a significant amount of in your daily diet. They are healthy fats that will not cause weight gain but can help keep it. The main sources for those fats can be found in:

Nuts

Fruits

Olive Oil

Canola Oil

Seeds

Fish oil

Flax seeds

Salmon, Herring, Sardines

Carbohydrates

According to USDA guidelines, a daily consumption for a healthy adult must comprise about half of the calories consumed during one day. If, for instance, you consume 1500 calories in total, then 750 of the calories must be derived from carbohydrates. Considering that each gram of carbohydrates provides the equivalent of 4 calories 187.5 grams of carbs are required to be consumed each day.

Similar to the fats in your diet, there's specific kinds of carbohydrates that are advised to consume and kinds to be avoided. This must also be taken into consideration when planning your diet.

Simple carbohydrates comprise a category of carbohydrates that should be avoided. The reason you should avoid them is due to the speed that they are processed. They are digested quickly, and they have directly impacting your blood sugar levels. The only time when they should be consumed is immediately after exercising as they can prove to be a quick energy source. If not, it's best to keep your consumption to an absolute minimal (they should not be eliminated completely in your food).

Complex carbohydrates are, however should be consumed since they require longer to digest. Here are the carbohydrate sources:

Potatoes, yams and beans

Brown rice (rice with the husk)

Fruits

Oatmeal

In essence, any whole wheat or whole grain products are an excellent source of carbohydrates.

The most important aspect to remember is the fact that neither of these three nutrients makes you overweight in any way. It is the total number of calories that come from the three nutrients that determines if you lose or gain weight.

Drinks

Let's now look at which drinks to consume and what drinks to avoid. It's not advised to drink calories in liquid form. While it's a simple way to consume calories however, liquids are not able to provide you with enough energy and you can feel hungry even after having the liquid. In this way your calorific intake is out of the norm and your attempt to shed weight fails completely.

Additionally, many soft drinks contain a high calories due to how much sugar they contain. Sugar is a basic carbohydrate and, as we've mentioned previously the carbs are to be kept away from. Therefore, avoiding them can help you lose weight, but also has an impact on your well-being. It also eliminates one of the major causes of weight gain through avoiding soft drinks.

However, fluids are not completely eliminated due to obvious reasons. Here are some drinks are safe to consume and those that are not. We will first take a look at drinks that we need to stay clear of:

Drinks to Beware of

A majority of drinks typically are consumed should be avoided from your weight loss plan. Soft drinks, sodas, and energy drinks, and other drinks need to be kept away from. Fruit juices should not be consumed as well. Instead, eat the actual fruit.

It is important to keep your intake of milk to an absolute minimal amount. While it's very nutritious, as we've mentioned earlier it doesn't give you a full stomach and you'll feel hungry quickly. In addition, alcohol consumption should be minimized (no alcohol consumption is best to be healthy as well).

Drinks that can be consumed

According to the report, there are only two drinks that are suitable for inclusion in a weight loss plansuch as green tea and water. It's not a surprise that water is among two fluids that make the list. The majority of human being's water is approximately 90% of blood in humans is composed of water. It is by far the most vital fluid can be consumed. It's calories are not there to be added to the other benefits of water.

There's no precise amount you can use to determine what amount of fluid that a person needs in a day. It's contingent upon a range of variables. Additionally, since water doesn't cause harm so it doesn't matter how excessive amounts in water (unless you're drinking huge quantities of water each day like 3 or 2 gallon!).

Chapter 4: Different kinds Of

Bodybuilding Supplements

Muscle building may not be as simple as you imagine it to be. If, for instance, you just lift weights and consume protein-rich food items it is possible that you will find your significant muscles hitting a stage of development. In this case, supplements could solve your issues. However, before you decide to spend money on the supplements readily available be aware of what kind of supplements will most likely be beneficial for you. This section of the book can to provide important details about this crucial issue regarding bodybuilding.

Hormonal supplements assist the natural hormones in your body in transmitting messages that prompt your body to act immediately.

Additionally, supplements can in the production of hormones, so your body is able to build stronger muscles. The two most important substances to induce this result are growth hormones and testosterone. You can increase the level of intake to the most possible levels, without having to take the risk of having a hospital visit as long as you speak with your doctor about the dose you need to consume.

Testosterone boosters can to increase the levels of this hormone in your body , so that you can gain larger, leaner muscle mass.

Testosterone is one of the hormones that naturally is produced by your body. It's purpose is to boost your muscle mass through improving the process of synthesis of the muscles proteins present within your body. It is good news if you're currently between the ages of 18 and age

35 testosterone boosters won't make much of an impact since your body already produces enough of testosterone (which your body eventually will utilize).

If you're over the age of 30 and have a lower level of testosterone, supplements won't boost your testosterone levels to overly high levels. However, they put your body into a state that can boost the amount of substance to its natural levels. When taking these supplements be sure ensure that you stay clear of areas that are polluted, soaps that contain triclocarban, high-sugar diets and stress. It is essential to adhere to this advice to stop your testosterone levels from falling.

Supplements with growth hormones are involved for helping you build big muscles.

Your body is able to naturally produce sufficient amounts of growth hormones. The name implies that it is the hormone an essential factor in the growth of cells and cell regeneration. It will gradually decrease as you age, and may contribute to making the physical appearance of your body appear to be synonymous with ageing.

If you do not make the switch to growth hormone use it is not possible to build muscles. The supplementation of this hormone could produce the same results as testosterone boosters. This means that you can boost your levels to the maximum natural levels if you're hoping to witness more muscle growth over a shorter amount of time. The intensity of your training and the age will determine if you are able to naturally produce more or less, of this kind of hormone. In this respect it might be more effective for the growth of muscle mass taking your supplements prior to go to bed.

Gaining more energy by taking a variety of energy supplements to aid in muscles training could assist you in gaining more strength in the training.

Due to this the muscle mass in your body will grow. The issue is that lots of energy-rich supplements can give you a an jittery feeling over the long haul. The majority of energy supplements are employed to help you shed some weight. To make sure that your supplement program isn't affecting your brawn-building goals that you have set You must adhere to the suggested list of supplements your doctor, trainer or dietician recommended for you.

Caffeine-rich supplements can help block various brain chemicals, that is a strong signal for sleep.

This may also cause that the heart beat at a higher rate, which increases the flow of blood to muscles as well as the size of the air passages. The research published in journals has shown that consuming caffeine prior to performing exercises that strengthen your body will increase the overall strength and allow you to complete even more numbers of repetitions. In essence, it gives you an added push you need to exercise even more. But, it is important to be aware that taking higher levels of caffeine in your system may result in an increased resistance to this substance. It is best to vary your intake of caffeine whenever you work out to the max.

Creatine is the result of methionine, arginine and Glycine.

The mixture of ingredients is regarded by many to be the staple of fitness enthusiasts. When you drink this mixture, you instantly get more ATP (adenine triphosphate). This is thought of as the body's main source of energy, but it is only the smallest amount within your body. This is the main reason why your main muscles are usually not able to perform during your last repetition.

Creatine helps in increasing the level of your muscles, so that you can do more repetitions in your training in resistance. In the long term this could result in more muscle groups that are stronger and larger. The muscles that are strengthened will largely depend on the muscles that you exercise during your workout exercises. In addition it can nourish the cells of your muscles. This will then improve the capacity to build more muscles and boost recovery. Studies have shown that creatine may aid in enhancing the capacity of the body to build muscle by about 14 percent in comparison to other compounds.

Chapter 5: Paleo With Intermittent Fasting

There's no better way to combine eating habits than the paleo diet with intermittent fasting. It's what the earliest humans ate and possibly Greek Gods too. Paleo foods include fish, meat fruit, nuts, and vegetables. It's what humans have eaten since the beginning of the time. It's been documented by the millions of generations that came before our time. Paleo is the oldest outline of what the human was meant to eat.

Combine that with intermittent fasting, and you'll soon be an modern-day caveman. Intermittent Fasting (IF) is the practice of not eating for prolonged durations of time. It is an eating time that is followed by a period of fasting which means you don't eat or drink something that contains calories. To get the most effective results, skip breakfast. You've been told all your time that breakfast should be the most nutritious meal of the day. however, this is utter nonsense. If you get up, you're energized because you've had a restful night sleeping. Your body is glowing with energy, but eating breakfast suffocates the natural energy. Instead of being bursting with energy, your body's taking energy to process the food you've eaten. Don't be a fool and take your breakfast off.

If you're building, you'll want your fasting duration to be shorter, and your eating interval to be longer. While you're chiseling, you'd prefer it to go reversed. IF is so effective that if you practice too much while building, you'll be unable to build any muscles. It's great when you're making chisels, however; it slices through every kilogram of fat that is in the body leaving your figure smooth as diamonds.

Here's what I personally do with IF. If I'm building, I'll leave breakfast out and that's all I do. My typical day is like this: I get up around 9 am and eat lunch at 12:15. I am able to have four hours of pure energy through me prior to eating during the day, leading to amazing productive mornings. I then eat three to four times more throughout the day to build up panty sweaty muscle. This is when I'm building. when I'm chiseling , it's like this: get up around 9am and eat lunch at 12. then eat around 6. I eat just twice every day while doing chiseling. These are massive meals that make me happy throughout the day. I take my food as seriously as a lion when working, a couple of large meals per day, and I'm satisfied.

Yesterday I had exactly as follows: at 12 noon 5 eggs that I scrambled as well as the avocado and a banana and lots of cashews. Then , for my second dinner of the day, an enormous seasoned steak, onions, some greens peppers, chicken and rice, and the peanut butter. That's what I normally consume. When I don't have cashews I prefer peanuts, almonds or any other variety of nuts. If I don't want to eat bananas, I prefer peaches, apples or any other type of fruit. If I don't like steak, I will eat deer, chicken, beef or lamb. There's always a replacement.

Create an IF / Paleo plan that fits into your lifestyle and not the reverse. Do not miss out on the fun of the world just to have your dinner.

Chapter 6: Diet And Nutrition For A Healthy Bodybuilder

Dieters and those who are trying to shed weight aren't the only ones affected by the new kind of diets that are introduced every year. With so many options, like low-fat, low carb, gluten-free etc. You can't determine if you should concentrate on protein only or a complete diet.

I can understand your dilemma I'm the same way once. Since I was constantly changing my diet, long-lasting results were difficult to achieve. I was eating for months before I noticed muscle growth. The issue is that the body was confused and wasn't sure how to so that it could take in the vital protein and nutrients it required to remain healthy and build muscle.

I stopped listening in on people who were bodybuilders or other bodybuilders and social media posts about diets. Instead I began to listen to my body, and then did studies to find out what diet or combination of diets could get closer towards my goals.

After hours of intensive research and a months into the new eating plan I began to see the results I'd been looking for.

A combination that promises success

A paleo-style diet and intermittent fasting as well as soup cleanse. Yes the combination of these three can do wonders. What is the way to achieve this? It's simple, we must first look at the features of each of the diets.

1. Paleo Diet

The paleo diet focuses upon eating meat which implies that it's among the most effective diets to give you the highest protein source. Contrary to a low- or no-carb diet it doesn't restrict carbs. It is a strict focus on the natural carbs found in fruits. If you do require more carbohydrates prior to or following training, you'll get them from fruits instead of artificial sweeteners.

The paleo diet is based on meat and is based upon the idea that our ancestors lived for around 140 000 years with no agriculture and their diet was dependent on the food they could gather or catch in the open air. Ten thousand years ago, when the first people began to settle and establish an established society agriculture was the main activity that allowed us to consume grain, consume milk past the age of infants, and eat foods that required cultivation to develop.

However, just 1,000 years are not enough for our genes to adapt to this style of eating and that's why we've become overweight and unhealthy. Our hunter-gatherer ancestors were strong and filled with energy. They prospered.

The paleo diet isn't an easy thing to remember. it's easy and wonderful tasty meals can be prepared. There are some tips to remember when following this diet:

It's a meat-based lifestyle However, it doesn't mean that vegetables aren't considered. Be sure to eat plenty of vegetables with every meal. Make sure to eat the vegetables that boost your hormones and help keep your hormones in balance so you will build lean muscles.

Your first meal must be a feast of fats and protein, not grains and carbs. Instead of eating cereal for breakfast for breakfast, as the first breakfast consume foods that are high in protein, such as bacon eggs or beef. You can also eat fish and other fish. This is a quick and easy casserole to make: steam some broccoli and cauliflower, shred it add 6 eggs and bacon, mix it all up and place it into a baking dish (shallow) to bake it for 30 to 45 minutes in an oven that is preheated.

Eat until you're no longer hungry. If you eat , and then stop and you're still hungry, you'll discover yourself opening your fridge every other minute to find something to consume.

You must ensure your meat consume is grass-fed and not processed.

The fish you consume should come from the wild

Eggs should come from grass-fed chickens.

No more food items that are processed

Say goodbye to sweet drinks

Limit your consumption of alcohol (especially beer, as it can increase estrogen) It is possible to have some wine that is dry.

2. Intermittent Fasting

Another famous diet that is more of an approach to life. It is possible to continue with the old way of eating, but include the. Intermittent fasting does not compare to starvation. It is simply a time when you don't consume food. You've decided not to take food, which means that you are fasting.

During this period of fasting there is no need to consume food or any calorific drink. It is only water or tea as the amount you'd like.

This kind of life style is practiced by a number of traditions which are still in existence such as the Muslims. They observe a fast from sunrise to the sunset over 40 days every year during Ramadan.

Intermittent fasting has been shown to be successful for all people who want to lose weight and build muscles. There are several methods of fasting that range starting from one that lasts 14-16 hours, to others which last for 36 hours.

Some people aren't able to sustain the long fasting and I am not one of them. This is the reason I chose to combine paleo eating and intermittent fasting , which lasts 14-16 hours. I practice this every day.

My last meal time is 7 pm and my next meal starts at 10:00 am until around 1:00 pm. I sleep around 11:00 pm. This implies that around the 8-hour fasting has passed while I am asleep. So, it's the most efficient method. 8 hours of rest, 2 hours of eating nothing before going to bed, and then the next when you wake upIt is very simple.

After that, my first meal (it isn't breakfast, hence why I don't call it breakfast) is full of proteins and fats that give me energy back. I take my food until I feel full. After about an hour I'm a fan of having fruits to help get healthy carbs into my body and I also get a few carbs by eating a couple of potato skin wedges.

Another benefit of fasting intermittently is the fact that it doesn't cause muscle damage; on contrary, you'll build stronger and faster.

3. Soup Cleansing

The presence of toxic substances is always present regardless of how hard we attempt to eat a healthy diet but the air remains polluted, as all other things are. All of it is absorbed by our bodies. This is why it's vital to cleanse your body at least every three months (with one week of soup cleansing) or once a month (a 3 to 4 days of soup cleanse) or just one day each week. It's all your choice.

If the body is stuffed with contaminants, it's unable to function effectively and inflammation, the only thing that can help fight injuries can actually begin to attack the body because the dirt that's collected confuses the body.

In a single soup cleanse it is crucial to drink only creamy soups that don't make your stomach require too much energy digesting. The focus is on energy in this case. The energy you generate won't be used to digest food, but your body will utilize this energy to cleanse itself.

Since you're on the paleo diet and intermittent fasting. The most effective time to cleanse your soup is every month for 2-3 days. If you are able to endure for 7 days eating only soup, do it (but at intervals of 3 months). If you're new to soup cleansing, it's acceptable to do it for just one day as a first step.

How to make an Bodybuilding Diet Plan

A lot of bodybuilders who are beginners as well as who have been around for a while know they require adequate nutrition to get the right look and weight for their muscles. But, even "experienced" bodybuilders aren't aware of how to develop the meal plan of their choice instead follow an established diet.

It wouldn't be simpler to stick to your own program? You could add food you love while still building muscles. It is best to plan your diet according to your obligations and stay away from building muscle. Of course, it's not always about training.

If you're spending the whole day in the gym but that doesn't mean you'll see results. it's because you're making sure that your muscles have the time to rest, and you aren't able to provide your body with the nutrition it requires.

What are the nutrients you require and in what amount?

While paleo is founded in not counting calories however when coupled with bodybuilding, it's essential to keep track of these. Not just the total calories however, you should also count protein, carbs, as well as fat.

Since I am not a fan of math (and many of you, too) so I won't be explaining how things are calculated. Why bother when you could simply locate an online calculator for calories. After you have decided about your calorie consumption then it's time to choose your macronutrient ratios which is Marco in short.

Marco is the blend of three essential nutrients your body requires to remain fit, healthy and build up muscles.

1. 10% carbs/50% protein/ 40% fat (most low-carb diets)

2. 50 percent carbs, 40% protein and 10 10% fat (not my current favorite however, it is still being is used by certain bodybuilders)

3. 40% carbs/40% protein/20% fat

I am not a fan of the percentages above because you must determine the appropriate protein intake based on your weight. It is 1g for every pounds. in body mass.

1. Vitamins and anti-oxidants. Vitamins are vital for muscle building However, I never

overlook fresh vegetables and fruits and opt for supplements instead. There are also essential trace elements found in vegetables and fruit that don't receive in supplements. It is essential to consume at least three or four fruits a every day, along with six or more cups of vegetables (the more you eat, the more). Take in colorful fruits such as prunes, grapes, and the berries. If you are eating vegetables, pick red bell peppers, kale as well as spinach. And make sure you include those that boost your testosterone levels.

2. What is fiber and why is it vital? It helps to lose the boring fat. The most appealing aspect is that each food that is high in fiber is low in calories, or has no any calories; yet, it makes you feel happy. It is essential to incorporate vegetables and legumes in order to obtain at minimum forty grams of fiber every day.

3. Omega-3 fats The body requires fats, particularly since it isn't able to produce these. It is crucial to get sufficient omega-6 and omega-3 each daily. The most effective sources include flax, mackerel and anchovies as well as herring, mackerel and salmon. Essential fatty acids not just help you build more muscles, but they can keep you fit particularly your heart. The body requires at minimum 5 grams of protein per every day.

4. Quality Protein - What did I not talk about protein before? Because the foods I mentioned in previous posts already contain a significant amount of it. If I had included chicken first before anything else, you could end up having more calories than the recommended daily consumption and you won't have the other vital nutrients. This implies that it's not only about chicken as protein sources are everywhere. It's even in large hamburgers,

however this is non-lean protein. You should focus on lean protein that comes from grass-fed animals.

Okay, so what are the foods that have the highest protein? Milk and eggs. And If you are able to tolerate lactose, choose milk. Keep in mind that beef isn't the most effective protein source. even quinoa contains more high-quality protein than beef.

5. Good Fats There are good fats for your body, and they shouldn't be overlooked and should instead be considered as crucial alongside other nutrients. Monoand poly-saturated fats are excellent for your health. Make sure to choose natural oils and not the liquid version. Consume nuts, olives, or avocados, and you'll take at 10% or more or more of the calories you consume from fats. In the past cholesterol was still seen as an evil

force, but not any more. Saturated fats should be derived from animals, and shouldn't exceed 5percent of your daily calories. Eggs are excellent to get this done, but you must be cautious because, when you eat eggs, you could easily overdo the recommended quantity.

If you choose to use eggs for protein It is crucial to consume only the whites (2-3 yolks are good). What is the bad fat? It is oil that has been cooked, and that's what is what all junk and snack food items contain...

6. Drinking water - Never neglect to drink your water. the body is made up largely of it. Without water, your body won't operate properly. It is essential to cleanse the body, and it is required to carry out chemical reactions, which include the building of muscles as well as energy production and burning fat. Like fats,

water also helps to lubricate joints. Water is not just a way to regulate the body temperature, but also aids in controlling appetite. If you are feeling hungry even after eating a large food, it could be an indication that you require more water. Water can help curb hunger and improve the metabolism of your.

I believe you understand my point. Use the daily calories recommended by your doctor to ensure you are getting all the essential nutrients. The minerals and vitamins you require for your wellbeing and hormonal balance along with protein, fats, and carbohydrates that give you the energy and motivation to exercise more to achieve the results you've been seeking. There's no way to tell you precisely what amount of calories, protein carbs, fats and proteins you need to consume with every meal or snack because everyone has their own demands for calories, and I cannot rely on all those exact nutritional values.

All in all, adhere to these three fundamental steps:

1. Follow the Paleo Diet

2. Include at least one days of fasting intermittently to achieve more rapid weight loss (a sixteen-hour fast)

3. Do a soup cleanse one time each month (for1-3 days) or at least once three times a year (a 7-day cleanse)

Chapter 7: Meet Your Body

Bodybuilding is about understanding your body's structure and how to shape, build and perfect every aspect of it. For that, you need to know your muscles. In this article we'll give you an overview of the major muscles of the skeletal system you'll be working with from the front to the back.

Front of Body

Shoulders (Deltoids) The shoulder is a three headed muscle with anterior, middle , and posterior sections. They are involved with each upper body motion when they are performing abduction and abduction (pulling shoulders away and towards to the human body). The deltoids also have the capability of rotation.

Chest (Pectorals) Pectorals: Two muscle groups make up the chest, the pectoralis major as well as the pectoralis major. The pectorals perform an adduction (pushing out of the chest) and medial rotation.

Biceps Brachii The Biceps Brachii has two heads of the biceps, the longer head as well as the short one. It can perform two functions - flexion at the elbow as well as supination of the elbow. Brachialis Brachialis is a muscle that extends from the ulna and the elbow. It aids in the elbow's extension.

Forearm (Brachioradialis) The primary function of the forearm is elbow extension.

Absdominals (Rectus Abdominis) The abdominals comprise of the rectus abdominalis, the external obliques, and an internal set of obliques. The rectus abdominalis is involved in the flexion and extension of the trunk. External obliques permit the trunk to flex laterally and the external obliques allow for lateral flexion of the trunk.

Thighs (Quadriceps) The rectus femoris is located across the mid-thigh area. It performs flexion as well as extension. The vastus muscles lie along either side of the femoris, and are responsible for the extension and flexion of legs. The adductors are located near the hip joint. They allow the lateral rotator to adduce, extension and medial rotation.

Calves The Gastrocnemius is the primary component of the calf muscles. Its role is to permit an ankle flexion. The soleus muscles lie below the gastrocnemius and on the opposite side that of your lower leg. It aids in the flexion of the ankle.

Back of Body

Trapezius It is the trapezius is located between the neck and shoulders, going all the way towards the bottom of your back. It is a way to increase the height of the scapula in addition to adduction and reduction of the scapula.

Lats (Latissimus Dorsi): The lats originate at the lower ribs, and are located on the medial aspect of the humerus. The muscle is responsible for the sought-after "V" form for the body's upper part. It is responsible for adduction, extension as well as medial rotation.

The Middle Back (Rhomboids) Middle Back (Rhomboids) Rhomboids are derived from the spine. They then extend to the scapula. Their purpose is to help in adduction of the scapula.

Lower Back (Lower Trapezius): The lower trapezius allows for a depressing of the scapula.

The gluteus medius, gluteus maximus and minimus allow for extension, lateral rotation , and abduction of the lower part of the body.

Hamstrings: The hamstrings comprised of the rectus-femoris the semitendinosus, the rectus femoris and the semimembranosus muscles. They are responsible for extension as well as flexion of the upper leg.

Chapter 8: the Biology Behind It All

As we've mentioned before many women are scared of lifting weights due to the fact that they don't wish to build up. It's a good thing that your female body simply not designed to build a mass of muscles! When you lift weights, it actually boosts the mass of your lean muscle. The more lean mass you possess and the greater amount of fat you'll be able to burn even if you're lying around. When you combine this with your body transforms into a fat-burning machine thus preventing you from having to become bulky.

If this isn't sufficient to convince you that you will not get bulky due to weight training consider your hormones. Women aren't producing enough testosterone to create a significant amount in muscle. In addition the majority of women don't consume enough calories to maintain an enormous muscle mass. Contrary to popular belief weightlifting alone will not automatically build bigger muscles. As we discussed in the previous chapter it is essential to consume food to provide your body with fuel. The bodybuilders who claim to be heavy have no idea what they are doing or are drastically altering their diet.

Once we've got that done It's time to focus on the most vital part in bodybuilding: your shape! As we said earlier, the beautiful women of this world are different in shape and sizes. Which one are you ? And how can you get to be the best you could be? This is the question we are on the lookout for. Find out what kind of person you are as well as what the recommended macronutrient ratios are!

Different body types

Ectomorph

Let us begin by acknowledging that not all people can be described precisely. Although you are able to pick out the majority of your traits however, the majority of people have some of the. The trick is to figure out one of the three main types you're most similar to for you to customize your diet and workout routine. Let's start with the smallest kinds.

If you're an ectomorph your body type will likely appear like an endurance runner. It is likely that you have a lower body structure with a smaller bone mass, smaller joints and have a high metabolic rate which results in slimmer body. A high metabolic rate is a sign that your body is able to take in more carbs! To calculate your macronutrients we recommend 50 percent carbohydrates 30, 30 percent protein as well as 20 percent of fat.

Mesomorph

If you belong to the mesomorph group and you are mesomorph, you will appear to be an athlete or bodybuilder! This type of body provides the ideal base to build muscle because your body is balanced and has the ability to maintain a lean physique and gain muscles. This type of body has a moderately sized bone structure, and is likely to look athletic. If you think you're in this type of body be sure to stick with an a ratio of macronutrients that is close to 40 percent carbohydrates 30 percent protein, as well as 30 % fat. Contrary to the ectomorphs that you are, your body cannot take on as much carbs. Instead, you should fuel your body by consuming protein in order to build the muscle!

Endomorph

At the opposite end on the spectrum is women who are an endomorph kind of physique. They are women who appear like powerlifters. They have a bigger bone structure, it also means that they have a larger body and more powerful than the majority of. Because of their size this type of body can perform better with a diet that includes more healthy fats and less carbohydrates. The macronutrients ratio recommended for women of this type of body is 25 percent carbohydrates 35 percent protein, along with 40 % fat.

As you can see, there's an explanation for why one diet doesn't work for everyone. After you've identified the type of body you're most closely related to, you'll be able to begin designing your diet around it. Naturally, every body requires various nutrients. When you're done with your day, the main goal should be eating healthy food for better results. We suggest cooking your own meals so that you can stay with the program. If you decide to eat out, make sure you keep your diet in mind to stay in the right direction!

Once you're aware of the nutrition that you should be putting into your body and body type is it time to move on there to check out the tools section. As your diet is likely to alter, the equipment for building your body may change based on what you're trying to achieve. Read on to discover which one is the optimal for you to see outcomes!

Chapter 9: The Preliminary Instructions

When we came up with the instructions for each exercise within our system Our goal was to keep the instructions as simple, concise and succinct as we can. Students should take the time to read each and every word of the instructions for each exercise prior to beginning the exercise. This is since we have noticed that there is a huge number of males and females who just glance at the drawing and believe it's enough. Each exercise is comprised of at least three or four elements (often several) that must be considered carefully. Illustrations are only able to show one aspect of the many that are required to complete the exercises This is the reason why it's so essential to study the instructions.

BREATHING. The pupil should breathe in sync with the movements. The proper way to breathe is this Inhale through the nose while you stretch the muscles. Then breath out with your mouth while relaxing the muscles. For example, do the regular Exercise No. 1: you breathe in while you bring the bell towards your chest, then you exhale as your lower the bell down to the hips. As you breathe, exhale forcefully. Don't actually blow, but make sure you get oxygen out of your lung. If you exhale and produce the sound "HA" that will assist you exhale properly.

Most importantly, DO NOT take a breath while performing heavy dumb-bell exercises. A lot of nonsense has been published and taught on the subject of deep breathing that lots of uninformed people are taught that when exercising, it's normal to take extremely long breaths and hold them for as long as they can. This is a complete misunderstanding. The role for the lungs are to remove carbonic acid from blood. If you are exercising, because the function of the heart gets accelerated as blood is pumped faster into the lungs. This means that your lungs have to perform quickly to remove the polluted air and provide the fresh air. Don't think by claiming that you are able to use a more effective method to breathe than the one we've outlined in the previous paragraphs. It's not true, and we should insist that you follow the guidelines we have provided in this regard.

Instead of holding your breath, we suggest to breathe in and out continually. When you are exercising, it is vital to open your mouth for complete oxygenation of the blood.

Bathing the Body

We suggest a warm bath over any other. We suggest a cold shower only for those who like these baths. Even in that case, we believe that the man should be strong and not overweight. A person who is overweight is likely to have better results when taking the hot tub. If you want to rest better and anxious people will benefit from taking a warm or hot bath prior to retiring.

Time to Exercise

We suggest that the workout be completed between 5 and 8 P.M. Or about 9:30 to 10 P.M. This assumes that you eat your dinner between 6 to 7.

Our experience has taught us that the greatest results from a heavy barbell exercise can be achieved by a person who exercises at least three to four times per week. If you are a beginner and not overweight, we'd recommend three times a week. People who are obese may gain from exercising almost every day.

In the event that any exercise is performed, the muscle tissue is destroyed and then replaced with fresh tissue supplied by blood. This process happens very quickly when heavyweight exercises are practiced. If a person is exercising using heavy dumbbells every day basis will increase quickly during the days when he is relaxing.

When a person is active each day, the exercise is no longer an enjoyable activity, turns into work. The weight of the dumbbell is so effective that its benefits will not be lost if an exercise session is skipped. If a person exercises every other day , he will come to exercise looking energetic and ready to get started.

If the above guidelines are followed , the bells must be used for between 30 and 45 minutes. There are many individuals, particularly boys who believe that they must exercise every day In this instance it is recommended that the workouts be divided into two segments. The first section should be completed every day, the second one the following day. The exercise duration shouldn't exceed 15 minutes per day.

Diet

My goal is to put my students in a position that they will take in food, digest, and gradually build up their regular diet. Personally, I believe that many of these diet trending diets are created for people who don't have the time to do enough exercise to stimulate appetite. It is possible that an overweight, over-fed businessman who performs none of his exercise will benefit in eating two meal per day instead of three and avoiding the most fatty foods, but I'm not sure how it's possible for an individual to build themselves up to a high degree by eating two meals per day, particularly if is exercising vigorously. The longer you run an engine, the greater amount of fuel it will require. If you drive a motor 40 miles per hour you'd be burning a large amount of coal than if running it at 20 miles per hour.

If someone is trying to strengthen himself by exercising He simply needs to eat enough food to replenish the tissue that has been damaged during exercise in addition, it is his responsibility to provide Nature by establishing a fund of to grow.

I've met hundreds of professional and amateur "Strong Men" but I can't find a single person who supports the two meals-a-day program. Also, I don't know anyone "Strong men" that are vegetarians.

Many of the men who are known for their strength consume three meals per day, they eat a diverse one, including eggs, meat, vegetables and cheese, fruits and more. I think a mix diet is the most beneficial for athletes.

I'm not saying that my students consume excessive amounts of pie, pastry or confectionery, consume too much alcohol or smoke cigarettes too often however I do think that the more they don't stress about their food choices, the more quickly they'll accumulate.

Tea and coffee are potent stimulants which is why they should not be consumed in excessive amounts. Milk is an excellent weight-loss product and it is feasible to gain a significant amount of weight through drinking milk even if you aren't exercising however, the weight gained by drinking milk without exercising isn't likely to be a solid flesh. Thin people are able to gain weight through drinking milk, and they could gain weight even faster when they drink beeror using malted-food products that are popularly advertised. The problem is that the alcohol consumption or malted drinks isn't an effective solid muscle. It is soft flesh which, instead of helping to make one healthier and more robust in any way, it simply adds weight for him to carry around. Not an extra muscle that can take a man's weight - it's a huge difference.

The same thing that has been spoken about tea and coffee can be applied to a larger amount to smoking, and particularly, to alcohol. Many athletes achieve greatness even though they are addicted to these substances, but never (cigarette or whiskey to the opposite, not ignoring) due to their use. The moderate use of these substances can not cause much harm, but be sure that they will do nothing to help. A healthy diet that is balanced with consideration of the needs of rest, and an established training program can bring out the best within the student.

Our nutritionists are always available to provide guidance for pupils who wish to reduce or increase their body weight in conjunction with their exercise. Fasting can be risky if taken under the supervision of a competent expert, and is it is not recommended otherwise.

In your routine exercises you will be provided with a routine with "increases;" that is the exercise is repeated several times. Beginning with a lower number of repetitions and with a lower poundage increasing gradually the repetitions until you reach your highest level, you increase the weight of your bell, and then begin with the MINIMUM number of repetitions.

In Exercise No. 1, you begin by doing five times. For Mondays and Wednesdays,, you repeat No. 1 five times. On Friday and Sunday 6 times on Tuesday and Thursday, seven times and so on until you're able to complete ten repetitions; after that, you will increase your weight by by 10 pounds. and begin again at five repetitions. You should be increasing one repetition every third day of your practice. (It is perfectly acceptable to do three workouts every week on the exact days each week instead of sticking strictly to the daily schedule of once every 48 hours. You can do Wednesday, Monday, Friday or Tuesday, Thursday and Saturday each week and get results that are completely satisfactory). For a variety of the program and "mixing up" barbell training and various other workouts, recommend to read carefully the guidelines in the 47th page, in the final paragraph, and also in the very first sentence on page 3.

This is also known in"the "Double progressive method" It is the most effective and efficient method to increase your muscle mass which builds muscle size quicker than lifting that weight on the bell just one or two pounds each week.

It's important to understand that nobody can maintain this growth for a long time. There will come an point at which the amount of repetitions is too much in relation to the weight you're carrying which means that the weight you're employing is now too heavy for you to for exercise, and you must perform the number of repetitions you have previously been able to do. You must then take on the NEW program consisting of "INCREASES". Instead of beginning at five repetitions and progressing until you reach ten, you should begin at three and progress to six. After that, you must increase the weight of your barbell to 5lbs. instead of 10 pounds. This is especially true for exercises number. 1 2, 3, and 4 of the Regular course.

Then you'll begin to increase in pounds and repetitions until you are unable to continue to progress with "increases". That is the moment to introduce a new method of exercise should be introduced that can take greater care to maintain the increase in strength that you have gained in order to continue your physical progress. Some students will wonder what the reason for this. The reason usually your body weight that sets the difference. A person who is heavier may use more weight in the course of training due to his body weight. There are also exercises are not recommended to place excessive weights in.

The goal of an exercise is to be an exercise. If you are doing body-building exercises it turns into a feat of strength, and is able to be performed only at least once then it is no longer useful in measuring the growth of muscles.

In Regular Exercises Nos. 6 7, 8 and 11 There is no reduction in number of repetitions is required, as these muscles will be bigger or a greater number of muscles is called an int action. In these exercises, the body weight of the pupil cannot control the limit of poundage utilized so quickly.

Chapter 10: Value of Meal Planning for Building Muscle

Planning and preparing meals is crucial not just for bodybuilders but also anyone who wants to change their physique! In nowadays, a lot of people, they depend to others for the preparation of their meals. They consume a lot of food out or eat out on the go and don't spend much time cooking their own meals as they simply don't have time or time!

If you're determined to build muscles fast and losing weight, or enhancing your performance in sports food preparation and planning must be the top priority in your daily life. When you do that you'll be sure that your eating habits will contribute to aiding you in achieving your physical goals.

As nutrition plays an essential part in any physical change, enhancing your nutrition habits will mean you have a greater chances of getting results.

When it comes to food preparation and planning, there are a few aspects you must be aware of. These are:

It is important to know what food items you can include in your meals

It is important to know the correct size portions

You must have necessary food available

It is important to take your time every day to cook your meals

Now, let's take a look at the following points:

You should know which foods you can include in your meals

It's obvious that you need to include healthy food choices in every meal you cook, but the definition of healthy differs between people.

In the end, when planning your meals, each meal should consist mostly of whole foods. This implies that they've undergone very little processing i.e. fruits and vegetables are great examples of foods that are whole. Chips or fries which are highly refined versions of potato do not belong in this category.

Of course, you should take a break from eating light baked or steamed vegetables but common sense has to prevail. Foods that are fried, packaged, or high-processed foods aren't suited to helping you reach your fitness goals, no matter whether you're trying to shed weight or gain muscles.

Every meal you eat must include a proportion of all three macronutrients (carbohydrate protein, fat and carbohydrate). Protein is especially important since it's the main ingredient of muscle tissue. But, that doesn't mean you have to ignore the other macronutrients. Fats perform a number of vital functions to the body. They also assist in boosting muscle-building hormones such as testosterone. It also aids in reducing your appetite, decreases the metabolism of carbohydrates and gives your body the energy needed to function.

Carbohydrates are essential to provide an energy source to your body, as well as serving as a fantastic "cell-volumizing" muscle-building agent.

When you're making meal plans here are a few examples of healthy foods for bodybuilders:

Protein food items: Steak chicken breast, eggs, fish beans, nuts, tofu and seeds, cottage cheese Protein powder

Carbohydrate foods: Rice, oats, sweet potatoes, pumpkin, peas, corn, fruits, milk, yoghurt, sauces

Fat foods: Oils, butter, avocado, nuts, seeds

A more complete listing of sources for food can be found in chapter 10.

It is important to know the correct size portions

Be aware of the correct portion sizes is crucial when planning your meals to give your body enough calories to support optimal performance, maintenance and/or development of the muscle tissues as well as not feeling hungry until the next meal. Proper portion sizes can also stop the body from eating excessive food intake, which results in a higher storage capacity of body fat.

The appetite you feel prior to eating can be a good indicator on whether your previous meal was of a sufficient amount or size. If the previous meal was too large , you are probably not feeling hungry in the least. But, on the contrary, if your previous meal was not enough, you'll probably be experiencing hunger long before the dinner!

You should have food items you require

Proper meal planning and preparation will ensure that the food you're planning to use in your meals is already on already in your kitchen and ready to cook. Although this may sound simple, it means that you'll have to buy your groceries from the grocery store or a store frequently. Thus, part of food preparation and planning is knowing what you'll need in terms of quantities, knowing how much you'll require for a given duration of time, like for a week, then taking it to the store!

Once you've started cooking your meals, the entire range of the ingredients you'll need will be in your pantry which makes the whole process quicker and less time-consuming.

You must take the time every day to cook your meals

The people who achieve the greatest results with regards to body transformation, whether it bebuilding muscle mass or burning fat from the body is those who establish the habit of regular, regularly scheduled meal planning and preparation. This means that they scheduled time every day, and usually the same time every day to cook their food for the next day.

Additionally, their meals during the day differ only a little and they consume the same food for every meal, day in and day out! Naturally, they might have a meal out or lunch or opt to bake a whole fish dinner instead of the usual meat or chicken served along with vegetables. But generally there's an incredible amount of consistency in the food that they consume.

While some might find this way of food boring, but if really want to build muscles and achieve the highest outcomes, it's an essential step to take!

If you like your food choices and indulge in treats from time to time There is no doubt that it could develop into a routine which will not only help your results improve and results, but be a significant step toward increasing your overall health and overall well-being throughout your life.

Chapter 11: Eating Well

If you've decided you'd like to start an exercise program for bodybuilding The effectiveness of the entire program can be greatly affected by the food you consume. Many people focus only on their workouts and don't pay at what they consume, even though it is an essential component of any fitness program. It is believed that the workout you do is only 30 percent of your bodybuilding 50% is ensuring you are receiving the right nutrition, and the rest is to ensure you have adequate rest.

The body is able to get energy from food. They are energy fragments that the body needs for work. When it comes to calories taking them in should not be the primary goal; it is far more vital to consume calories that can provide the most benefit to your exercise.

You'll need energy to do your exercise each day. This energy is derived from many diverse nutrients. Carbohydrates are one of the most essential ones.

Carbs

The body receives the highest quantity of glucose through carbohydrates. It is a basic carb which your muscles and liver store as glycogen. It is the primary source of energy stored in your muscles. Your muscles are full and appear good when they have glycogen in their storage.

It is also an energy source for your brain, and also for the production of blood in the body. Since glucose is made of proteins, the body protein within the muscles needs to be broken down before. If you aren't getting enough carbohydrates in your diet the body will break down muscles to make glucose.

Thus, carbohydrates should comprise the largest part of your caloric intake every day once you begin a bodybuilding program. Take advantage of the natural complex carbohydrates like oatmeal, potatoes and brown rice, sweet potatoes and whole grains of breads.

Complex carbohydrates that are not processed are created through long chains of sugar which take a considerable amount of time to be digested. This is why they encourage regular blood sugars. This assists in counterbalancing the fatigue and exhaustion. It also helps to release insulin, the principal anabolic hormone produced by our body.

For men, multiply the body weight by 3. The result will be the amount of carbohydrates in grams you should incorporate into your daily diet. For instance, a 200 pound man needs to take in 600 grams of carbs every day. For women take your weight and multiply it by two. This figure will tell you the amount of carbohydrates you consume daily in grams. For example women need to have 250 grams carbohydrates each day if she weighs around at least 125 pounds.

Alongside carbs, your diet must include sufficient fibre too. Fibre boosts sugar and amino acid uptake as well as promotes the development and the growth of glycogen within muscles. This makes the muscle more at ease with anabolism. Two of the best sources of fiber are beans and oatmeal.

Reduce your carb-based meals into six portions over a day. This method is more practical and encourages the continuous release of insulin which triggers an anabolic or muscle-building state. Indulging in too many carbs at once isn't an ideal choice because fat-storing enzymes are activated, and you get rid of the "hard" appearance of muscle.

Take advantage of the simple carbs and eat them right after your exercise. Simple carbs like honey, sugar and refined food items can be digested quickly and easily. Consuming carbs after exercise will increase anabolism and prevent catabolism. Consuming simple carbohydrates can increase fat storage , especially if you've not exercised.

There are fewer chances that carbohydrates will be stored as fats if you include the carbs in your post-training meal. The reason is that carbohydrates are able to replenish glycogen levels before they can increase the storage of fat. It is a good idea to consume around 25 percent of the total carbohydrates in this dish.

It is well-known that breakfast is without doubt the most crucial breakfast during the course of the day. So, aside from the post workout meal breakfast is the ideal moment to consume carbohydrates. Because of your fast overnight the levels of glycogen in your muscles and blood sugar levels are lower early in the morning. Your body needs to replenish those levels prior to the fat storage process is activated.

The amount of carbohydrates you consume should decrease with the passing of time. The body won't require more carbs since the energy requirements decrease also. This is the reason why if you consume more carbs at night your body may start taking them in as fats and you could gain weight instead of mass.

If you are looking to build up your muscles while losing fat, it is recommended to shift your intake of carbs. Bodybuilders are more likely to shed fat when they rotate their intake of carbs as opposed to those who maintain the same amount of carbs while eating a diet.

For example for a bodybuilder who weighs 200 pounds may be able to alter the amount of carbs consumed each day, rather than eating 600g each day. Consume 300 grams over two days (50 percent less) followed by the normal 600g for two consecutive days, and then 900g (50 percent more) over the next two days.

Although the overall intake is the same as before, the new timing could work better as it decreases glycogen levels in muscle during the initial two days (to encourage the loss of fat) Then the levels of insulin will rise on the last two days to make sure there is no losing muscle. For bodybuilders who aren't as athletic, carb rotation may provide exactly what they want reduced fat and not losing muscle.

Protein

Protein is another vital nutritional element that every bodybuilder requires. Amino acids are thought as the primary proteins' building blocks, similar to glucose molecules, which are the carbohydrates' building blocks.

Protein in our bodies is the main ingredient responsible for the growth and healing of tissue. Proteins are the building blocks of our body's structure.

For bodybuilders, one important aspect of protein metabolism is the nitrogen balance. Nitrogen balance is the difference between how much nitrogen that is taken in and the amount lost. In the event that your loss of nitrogen is greater than what you absorb the body will break down muscle tissue to equalize the nitrogen loss. In contrast when the intake of nitrogen exceeds the amount of nitrogen you lose it will put you in a condition of muscle growth (since the nitrogen you have left is used to construct muscles).

The intake of protein can be directly related to nitrogen levels in your body. The principle that was mentioned earlier applies to protein intake, too. If the protein intake is higher than the output, nitrogen levels are maintained by promoting muscle development. This is precisely the thing you want when you are a bodybuilder.

If you have a nitrogen imbalance that is in negative the body is constantly decreasing the body's protein and muscle. The consequences of this can be evident in those who are in pain, hungry or suffering from a fever. This is called the catabolic state. Catabolic is a state of the body which the compounds are continuously broken to provide energy. In the bodybuilding world catabolic is the term used to describe loss of muscle.

However when your body is in a nitrogen balance positive, it's in anabolic mode. This is different from catabolic as the substances (proteins) join to form muscle tissue. In anabolic the growth of muscle is accelerated and this is the reason it is essential for bodybuilders to maintain an equilibrium of nitrogen.

The most effective way to maintain your body in an the state of anabolism involves eating approximately the exact quantity of protein (in grams) as you weigh. So, an athlete who weighs 150 pounds would need to consume 150g of protein every day. When you're thinking about what you should eat to meet your daily protein requirements take into consideration food items that provide a complete source of protein like eggs, meat and fish.

Another question that is frequently asked is, what do I do if I am currently on an eating plan? If you are on a diet while building muscle, your protein intake can be increased to as much as 1.5 times your body weight. This is due to the fact that you cut down on the intake of fat and carbs while dieting, which means that your body is burning more protein in order to supply energy which would otherwise be given by other nutrients.

For your convenience in your protein intake Here is a reference for the content of proteins in a few commonly consumed foods:

Foods containing protein

5 ounces of beef 35g of protein

5 ounces tuna , 43g of protein

5 ounces roasted ; roasted chicken contains 43.5g of protein

1 egg contains 6g of protein.

1 cup milk has 8g of protein

One tablespoon of peanut butter contains, 9g of protein

Two slices of cheddar, 14g of protein

2-slices of Whole Wheat Bread with 5g of protein

1 cup of cooked broccoli with 5g of protein

1.25 cups of beans contains 15g of protein

Though some might argue that eating a lot of protein is bad in terms of health and fitness, it's important if you plan to exercise hard regularly. The amino acids present in protein provide an energy source essential to help you build your body on a regular routine. Be aware that your protein balance must always remain positivity (anabolic) rather than positive (catabolic).

Fats

The first question to mind right now was: what do fats have to relate to bodybuilding? Fats are a vital nutrient that provides the energy and nourishment required for working out. The fats combine with glucose in your body to supply energy. It also stops degrading proteins (for energy) that promotes the growth of muscle.

There are two kinds of fats: saturated and unsaturated. Saturated fat is considered bad while unsaturated is a good fat. Your aim? Beware of the bad fats. Saturated fats are a major cause of the development of high levels of cholesterol as well as heart disease since they aren't readily broken down by the body. These fats are typically discovered in products from animals, such as cheese, meat, milk and egg yolks. Seafood is another source of saturated fats.

These saturated fats raise the levels of cholesterol called high-density lipoprotein (HDL) and low-density lipoprotein (LDL) within the body. While HDL is beneficial for us, more elevated levels of LDL may cause heart diseases because they block the arteries. They're also more difficult to break down, and they are quickly retained as fat that ultimately leads to weight gain.

Trans-fats present in processed food products that are commercially produced must be avoided as well. They remain more time in our bodies, and can cause our immune system function more quickly.

This can cause diabetes, stroke and heart disease. To stay healthy and increase muscle growth, remove all sources of trans-fat in your diet.

Now, the main issue is what is it that makes unsaturated oils "good"? Unsaturated fats are chemically more complicated than saturated fats. This allows them to be easier to breakdown to the body. Certain unsaturated fats work as antioxidants and help to reduce the amount of fat tissue within our bodies (promote the loss of weight). They can be found naturally in nuts and in fruit like avocados. Unsaturated fats are a great positive impact on cardiovascular health because they decrease LDL (also called "bad cholesterol") levels within the body.

If you're unsure whether your favorite snack is made up of saturated and unsaturated fats You can determine it by looking them up! At the temperature of room unsaturated fats exist in liquid forms like oil, and saturated fats are hard and solid.

Therefore, the general rule for fats isto avoid animal lard, and utilize oils like canola and olive oil. Be aware of the amount of fat in processed foods and make sure that the amount of saturated fats remains at a minimal amount.

There's a particular kind of fat called Omega 3 Fatty acids, that are considered to be the top fats to include included in the diet of your. The Omega 3 fats are found in fish and offer remarkable health benefits. They help reduce inflammation, improve the function of your brain, as well as stop the growth of cancerous cells within the body.

Additionally Omega 3 Fatty acids can also help combat joint pain, depression and fatigue, as well as diabetes. They are great for building muscle because they promote recovery of the muscles which is vital in the'rest' phase when you are working out. Fats are a vital component of every diet. They play an essential function in protecting the vital organs within our bodies. They give us the energy needed to complete the daily chores, and offer us the sensation of fullness after eating.

A healthy diet rich in fats isn't only essential to maintain good health, but it can help you stay healthy and strong as well! Be aware that eating too much of something can be harmful for your health. This is the reason I've provided some tips to help you keep your fat intake healthy:

*Use olive oil while cooking (and for salad dressings).

Try substituting lunch meats with tuna and avocados in your lunches.

Instead of chips, eat peanuts (no more than 1/2 cup).

Increase the quantity of fish included in your diet. Consume fish meals at least 3 times per week to increase the amount of Omega 3 intake.

Eliminate all sources of trans fat such as fast food and commercially processed food items,

*When baking, sprinkle with nuts and seeds instead of candy or chocolate.

As I stated in the previous chapter eating a healthy diet is an crucial aspect of any fitness program. You must pay close focus on what you're doing and eating. That includes alcohol too. Being a bodybuilder drinking alcohol may cause a negative impact on your development.

Alcohol is basically empty calories. It has no nutrition, there is no proteins, no fats and there are no carbohydrates. However, it does contain high levels of calories, which reduces metabolism in the body and reduces its capacity to digest food. Also, it encourages weight gain, which is not beneficial for bodybuilders.

Another reason to avoid drinking alcohol is because it slows the growth of muscles. The effects of drinking after a night out will decrease you're exercise and it also decreases protein production (the process by which muscles are created) by more than 20 percent! There are two reasons alcohol reduces protein synthesis.

The primary reason is that alcohol can dehydrate the body, and in particular the muscles cells. Dehydration can trigger a catabolic atmosphere which ultimately leads to the loss of muscle rather than growth. The reason for this is that alcohol prevents important nutrients like iron, calcium and potassium from being into the body. This hinders the relaxation of muscles and growth.

Alcohol also boosts hormones in the body and reduces testosterone levels. More testosterone levels make it ideal for an intense exercise, however because alcohol decreases testosterone levels testosterone levels, you can lose the intensity in your weight-training.

So, it is suggested to stay clear of drinking alcohol at all cost. The most beneficial way to protect the body is consume a large amount of water. Water is vital to every process that happens that occurs in your body. It increases the metabolism of your body and improves blood circulation.

The majority of doctors and experts suggest drinking eight glasses of water every day to maintain your health. For bodybuilders, this number is significantly higher. It is because you are dehydrated rapidly during workouts and need to make up for it. Bodybuilders should consume at least half a gallon water every day. However, tea and coffee drinks as well as soda are not recommended as they cause dehydration, as opposed to drinking water.

It also assists in cleansing the body. It eliminates toxins and metabolic waste from the body , thereby promoting digestion. It also eliminates excess ketones, nitrogen and Urea. Additionally, water is essential for kidneys to function well. In the absence of sufficient water, the burden shifts from kidneys onto the liver. The liver stores non-processed fat as energy. As the liver is performing its kidney's functions and burning less fat, which will eventually, this will result in weight gain.

In addition, water is also vital in shedding that excess weight of water. This is because when we take in less water, the body believes that there is water in short supply. This is why it stores excess water within the cellular space in the body. This makes the skin appear thin and soft. If you consume plenty of water your body doesn't require any unnatural actions and, therefore, doesn't keep it in cell spaces.

Water is also an essential ingredient that supplements must work. Supplements like creatine function because they draw water into the muscles , increasing their growth. This is the reason you have to make sure that your water intake remains in the right amount throughout your bodybuilding routine.

A healthy diet is crucial to an effective fitness program. If your diet is not healthy regardless of how much you train or how long your workouts are, you won't get the results you want to see. Here are some general guidelines to help you meet your nutritional needs in your bodybuilding routine:

*Drink skim milk or soy milk

Use artificial sweeteners in place of sugar.

*No soda, coffee or tea.

There is no fast food in particular pizzas and hamburgers. They are only a source of bad fats and do not contain nutritional value.

* Consume plenty of fish daily to boost the levels in Omega 3 fats.

*Chicken breasts and veggies are an excellent addition in any diet.

Take a close look at the nutritional information on the labels of processed foods. Remember that you must stay clear of saturated fats.

*During the course, at a minimum limit the amount of fruit you consume (except avocados). While they are healthy and healthful, they could be detrimental to your exercise.

Do not skip meals, but you can transform three big dinners into smaller meals. This will prevent your body from entering "starvation state."

Our body's ability to adapt is astounding. Although you may face some issues with your new diet plan at the beginning, after your (and the body) have become used to it, you'll never be thinking about the unhealthy food choices!

In the next chapter we'll look at sample meal plans to eliminate any doubts regarding the right time and food choices.

Chapter 12: Exercises to build muscle at Home

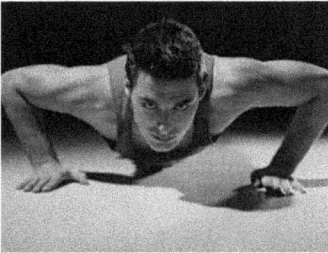

There are numerous reasons to build muscle through working out at home rather than going to the gym. Many of us work in jobs that require an enormous amount of energy and time, so many of us don't even have the ability to attend a gym due to inability to find the time or energy. Most people don't have time to go to the gym and work out for around an hour and return to home. Additionally, exercising at the convenience of your home can help you save on gym costs and membership fees.

At home , you can do dumbbell exercises and gravity workouts to achieve the toned and muscular body you've always wanted. It is possible to do these every day to increase your the strength and endurance. The first thing we will discuss is the exercises.

Different types of Bodybuilding Exercises

Warm-up Exercises

Prior to and following every session of strength training Make sure to do 5- 10 minutes of cardiovascular and stretching exercises. This can serve as your warm-up and cool-down periods.

Exercises for Gravity

A majority of us have minimal or no equipment for exercise at home. It is possible to use gravity and the forces it draws us to exercise different parts of our bodies. The exercises in the book consist of compound exercises which work different body parts simultaneously that makes your workout less time-consuming but still as vigorous. If you adhere to strictly, you're sure to reap the benefits of these exercises.

Exercises with dumbbells

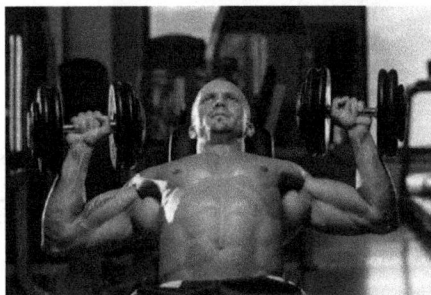

The right weight for dumbbell exercises is essential to getting the best outcomes. A weight that is too light can cause you to lose time, and the wrong weight could cause injury. Utilizing a lighter weight to practice and learn proper form before lifting heavier dumbbells gradually. Be sure to follow the correct form to avoid injury.

Bodybuilding Exercises at home

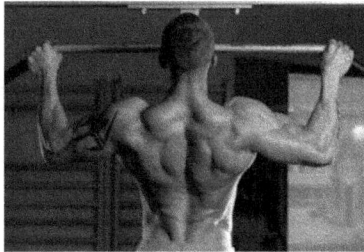

The following workout routine for strength is designed to be used for working out at home. You can pick it up at the beginning. The program includes a warm-up workout as well as a gravity workout. It also includes a dumbbell exercises. It's specifically designed to focus on the major body part within the course of a single day. Based on your fitness goals, you may decide to mix and match workouts into your workout. Let's begin the exercise to give you that muscle-toned, toned body.

Warm-up Exercises

These exercises can serve as warming-up and cooling-down routines.

High Knees

Keep your posture straight and place your feet the shoulder width. Then, lift your knees one at a time toward your the chest. Then, quickly return your feet to the floor. This exercise should last for one minute.

Jogging in Place

Take your feet of the floor and simulate running in the same spot for two minutes.

You can increase the speed and raise your knees up for greater level of intensity.

Stretching

Do a thorough stretch of your arm as well as your back, chest and thigh muscles, as well as hamstrings, the hip and calf muscles prior to exercise for strength.

Upper Body Exercise

Push-ups

Start by facing the floor with your legs joined. Hands should have about 2 inches larger than your shoulder width and slightly higher than the neck line. For this to be done correctly the back must always be straight , and your elbows point toward the sky.

You should push your body upwards, and gently lower it. Don't go all the way down, to keep the muscle tension. The muscle you want to target is the chest . However, your shoulders, triceps as well as back muscles are receiving some exercise to stabilize muscles.

Be sure to breathe through the workout. Breathe in as you go down, and exhale on your climb up. Perform 10 - 15 repetitions for each set, and at least 3 sets. Pause for 1 minute between sets. Increase the amount of reps you do as you get stronger. To build maximum muscle the last reps must be challenging to finish.

Pull-Ups

If there is a structure at your home or have a solid base, this exercise will be ideal for getting an expansive and supple back and also working your shoulders as well as your biceps for stabilizing muscles. It may be difficult for those who are trying it at first, but the amount of repetitions will gradually increase as you get grasp of it.

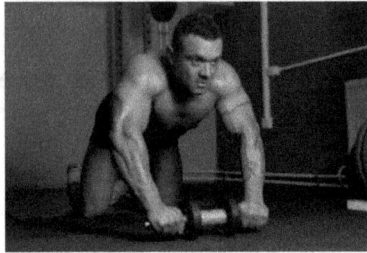

Set your hands approximately two inches more than the shoulder width on both sides with your palms facing forward. Slowly raise your body till your head is the same height as your hands. Slowly reduce your weight. Some people bend their knees for better stability.

Inhale as you go down, then exhale after exploding upwards. Other people do it in reverse, since that they are lowering their body more slowly. If you're looking for more "pump" it is possible to do it, but for those who are new, I recommend you increase you strength before doing it.

Alternations can be created by changing the positions of your hands (for instance, you can place your palms in front of the face) or by placing certain weights to your lower back. Perform as many pull-ups as you can in a single set and at least 3 sets.

Dumbbell Press

It can be done on a flat or inclined bench, provided that you you are using dumbbells with the correct weight. Be sure to keep your elbows straight and keep the dumbbells up to the top.

This is an excellent isolation exercise to build determination and endurance to your back. It also allows you to isolate the outside pecs through lowering your dumbbells down to the point where the weight rests on your shoulders. Do 10-12 reps for each set, and 3 sets is the minimum.

Arm Exercises

Dumbbell Tricep Overhead Extensions

This exercise lets you utilize a dumbbell to exercise your triceps one step at a time , or you can make use of both hands to grasp the dumbbell.

The method remains the same , despite every variation. Make sure your elbow(s) are always directed towards the ceiling. allow the dumbbell to touch you on the inside of your neck lightly before returning it to the starting position. Do 10-12 reps for each set, and at least 3 sets.

Dumbbell Kickbacks

Maintain your spine straight, and keep your arm in extension for around one second before lowering it. This helps your triceps develop that extended burn you're trying to pump. Do only one rep on the one side prior to shifting to the opposite side. By switching sides, one is able to relax a bit while another side is in the process of working.

Perform 10-12 reps for each set and perform 3 sets at a minimum.

Dumbbell Curls

The dumbbell curl is an exercise with multiple variations, yet it produces basically the same outcome. Even those who don't exercise know how to perform the dumbbell curl, but there are a few aspects that you should be aware of in order to get it done correctly.

If you're performing an alternate curl with a dumbbell do the first turn on one end prior to starting with the next. Most people begin to curl one arm , while the other is moving downwards. This doesn't allow you to increase the power. Also, don't lean back too much and make sure you don't "roll" your shoulders.

Perform 10-12 reps in each set and 3 sets for a minimum of.

Shoulder Exercise

Side Lateral Raise

The lateral raise comes in many variations, including an alternate front raise as well as the bent-over lateral raise , but the most well-known version is the side lateral raise. The dumbbells must be placed on your sides and must be raised to approximately shoulder height without bent elbows.

Be sure you aren't leaning back when lifting the weight. This is normal in the beginning when you put the dumbbells on the floor instead of having one dumbbell per side. It can be a good idea since it makes it easier to keep the perfect posture.

Perform 10-12 reps for each set, and at least 3 sets.

Core Workouts and Abdominals

Crunches

For abdominal strength, perform some crunches, as illustrated below.

Be sure to don't lock your fingers in order to avoid pulling your neck upwards, which puts stress on your neck muscles rather than the abdominal muscles. Also, you don't have to lift your neck all up (military fashion) as it can cause injury to your lower back.

Plank

Another excellent abdominal workout involves the plank. Simply keep in the plank for around 30 seconds at a stretch and you will be working your midsection, and possibly some in your deltoid muscles.

You can increase the duration when your resistance improves or try different variations of this workout.

Dumbbell Side Bend

The side bend of dumbbells strengthens your core and abdominal muscles. The key to the exercise is to maintain your back straight and only bend at your waist. Begin by holding a dumbbell in your right hand. Then, bend to the right as much as is possible. After that, return to the starting position and then bend towards the left side as much as you can before returning to your starting position.

Following 10-12 repetitions, swap the dumbbell back to one hand, then do the same with your other and continue. Do 3 sets at a minimum.

Ab Roller

A roller for abs can provide you with athletic ab exercises. Place your knees on the exercise mat and place an ab roller with your hands, putting them below your shoulders, in a push-up position.

Slowly move forward and then draw away from the roll. Be careful not to hold your hands out too long so that you can't turn your body back. Don't allow your back to slide.

Complete 12-15 rollouts for each set and three sets at a minimum or as per your level of fitness. Alternations can be made by stretching your rollouts or by tying a band for resistance on your fingers.

Lower Body Exercise

Squats

This is an excellent exercise to strengthen or tone your legs. This can be accomplished using a pair of dumbbells, barbells with weights as well as a water jug an exercise vest that is weighted or your body weight. It is not just for the legs but can tone the midsection, too.

Your feet should be approximately shoulder width apart. While keeping your lower back straight then slowly bend your knees to the point that your knees sit above your thighs. Don't move your body too far forward and ensure that you keep your eyes up as you go down in order to maintain your balance.

Inhale as you go down and exhale while you climb towards your starting position. Perform the minimum of 15 reps for each set of 3 to 4. This workout is sure to bring your body back to balance that is lacking in the majority of people, not just those who exercise frequently.

Calf Raises

There aren't much more in bodybuilding that are more impressive than a big hip and a twig an lower leg. If you're working your legs, be sure to exercise your calves, too.

Find a set of dumbbells. Stand on a platform , keeping your feet's heel in the air. Lift your entire body up a small amount, then slowly lower it back to the ground. Do 10-12 reps for each set and 3 sets at a minimum.

This tiny movement can assist you in getting that stunning pair of calves that will go with your thighs that are slender.

Jumping Jacks

The majority of us are aware of that jumping jacks are a thing and have performed them when we were young. This workout is perfect to work the glutes, hip flexors and the quads. It also targets calves, abs and shoulders, as well as hamstrings and hamstrings. stabilizing muscles.

It's a fantastic aerobic and anaerobic workout that increases strength and endurance while simultaneously. Simply do 50 repetitions for each 3 sets. This is an excellent way to finish for your workout routine.

A 7-Day Training Program

The following is a seven-day plan to begin with to increase strength and build lean muscles. The program will focus on a important body part each day, then rest on Wednesdays and Sundays.

Monday: Upper Body

Tuesday Core and abs

Wednesday: Rest day

Thursday Friday: Arms

Friday Shoulders

Saturday The lower body

Sunday: Rest day

Chapter 13: Activities

You might not be familiar with certain terminology used as part of exercising. In the same way it is important to know what specific exercises are and how to safely complete these.

There is a variety of tasks you can take part in and so many in reality there isn't enough space for publishing every single one. Whatever the case, a course lessons in the basics can be a huge help.

Dumbbell Bench Press

Place yourself on the edge of a comfortable seat with the dumbbells resting in your knees. In one swift movement then roll over onto your back and carry the dumbbells to an angle slightly away from your shoulders or even further. Your palms should be facing your movements.

Turn your elbows around 90 degrees with your arms in a straight line with the floor. Push the weights upwards with your chest in a triangular motion until they cross with the middle line that runs through your entire body.

While lifting, concentrate on observing the weights that have been that have been adjusted and. The same approach is used when you are descending.

Standing Military Press

In this workout you'll need barbells. Maintain your legs around shoulder width apart and raise the barbell up to your chest.

Bolt your hips and legs while keeping your elbows some distance below the bar. Push the bar until it is an appropriate distance above your head.

Lower the ringer down to your chest's upper part or to your jaw, based on what is most comfortable to you. The exercise can also be done with dumbbells, or on the weight bench.

Pushing Lying Triceps

Set up on a level bench using a twist bar in an overhand grip. Relax your back until the top on your back is level with the edge of the seat.

When you're lying down as you lie back, raise your arms above your head to ensure that the bar is easily removed from your eyes. Make sure your elbows are tight and your upper arms firmly in place throughout the workout.

The key to this exercise is to keep your arms in a relaxed posture. Slowly lower the bar until it's almost touching your forehead.

Lift the bar back with a gentle, clear bend like motion. In the direction of the entire, you should bolt your elbows completely.

SIDE TERRAL Dumbbell Raise

Sit upright, with your feet spaced from each other and your arms positioned next to your body. Put a dumbbell into each hand, with your palms turned toward your body.

Maintain your straight arms and then lift the weights up and to the sides until they are barely higher than the bear level. Then slowly let them fall back towards your side.

Keep your palms pointing toward the floor as you raise the dumbbells , with the intention that your shoulders are lifted instead of your biceps complete the required steps.

Be sure to lift the dumbbells upwards instead of moving them upwards. Make sure you don't lean forward as you do this, or else you could cause injury on your spine.

Minister Curls

This exercise is best completed by using a unique twist seat for evangelism however, you can also do this without this by doing some adjustments.

You should sit towards the top of the seat that is weighted, and then place something on your lap such as the firmest pad or few cushions beneath your arms in your lap.

Take the twist bar in your hands facing upwards. Do not slouch on the cushion. Sit in a straight position.

Utilizing the shoulder's width grip to grip the bar with two hands. Turn the bar upwards with a bent. Be careful not to shake or swing to move the bar.

The muscles should be used for lifting the weight. You should not use push. The purpose of this workout is to build biceps.

Transfer the bar to your desired level, ensuring that the obstacle is most notable at the beginning and end.

Reduce the bar slowly, working the muscle that is moving down. You could also use dumbbells to exercise on one arm at any time.

Situated Dumbbell Curl

You should sit towards the end of a chair and place your feet on the ground. Make sure you keep your back straight, and your head straight.

Begin by lifting the dumbbells from an appropriate distance. Keep your palms towards the ceiling. Turn the weight upwards and twist your wrist until they are over your hips.

Do your biceps press at your highest and then slowly decrease the weight.

Do not lift the dumbbells up and then bring them back up as you work those muscles! You can perform this exercise while standing, however the sitting location will help you avoid unintentional behavior.

One-Arm Dumbbell Row

Begin by placing your right feet on the floor , and your left knee resting on a flat seat. Lean forward to support the weight of your abdomen by placing your left arm sitting on the seat.

Your back should be in a straight line and roughly parallel to the floor.

Get down and grab the dumbbell using your right hand. The left arm should be secured to the elbow in order that it can support the abdominal region.

Before starting, you should look straight ahead instead of looking on the floor, so you can keep your back straight. Make sure your abs are in place to prevent your body from moving to the side when you lift the dumbbell.

Make sure you pull your elbow back as far you can. The dumbbell should be in a manner that is parallel to your middle.

After you've pumped the dumbbell up to until you're able to gradually lower it to its original position. Change arms after one set.

Dumbbell Shrugs

Make sure you are standing straight with your feet in a bear's width. Do two dumbbells while keeping your arms hanging by your sides.

Then, you can hang your shoulders for a long time. Bring your shoulders up until you can , and then slowly return to the starting position.

It is also possible to rotate your shoulders by going upwards in a circular motion in a back-to-front movement, and afterward, retrace them. It is also feasible using the barbell.

Standing Calf Raises

This is possible using the use of a specific machine in an exercise facility or that can be adjusted to work with no machine.

You can face a wall by placing your body in front of the divider. Place your palms pressed against the divider, and your feet at a level with the floor.

Maintain your posture and gradually raise your soles of your feet to the point that you're at the tips of your feet.

Keep the constriction tight and before slowly returning to the original position, with your feet firmly to the ground.

Crunches

Lay flat on your back, with your feet firmly on the groundor on a chair with your knees bent to 90 degrees. If you're laying your feet on a chair, place your feet about 3 to 4 inches apart and then point your toes inward so that they meet.

Place your hands lightly on the opposite sides of the head, keeping your elbows inside.

Do not put your fingers in your head!

Then, push the little muscle of your withdrawal into the floor to break your muscle strength. Start rolling your shoulders away from the floor.

Continue to push down as fast as you can using the lower part of your back. Your shoulders ought to rise from the floor about 4 inches. Your lower back should stay at the level of the flooring.

The spotlight is for moderate and controlled growth Do not rip off yourself by using energy!

Dumbbell Hammer Curls

With the dumbbells in both hands Keep your arms by your sides and your palms face one another. Keep your elbows locked into your sides. Your elbows and abdominals should be in the same spot throughout the entire exercise.

Keep your palms in front of each other. Twist the weight of your right hand in a semi-hover towards your left shoulder.

The biceps should be pressed hard at the top of the lift, and then slowly lower the bar.

Make sure you don't twist your wrists while you exercise! It is also possible to complete an arm at a time, and also switch arms.

Slope Dumbbell Press

Place yourself on the edge of the sloping seating set approximately 45 degrees. Put a dumbbell into each hand and set them on your legs. Then, taking each at a time will raise them to your shoulder height, as you push your back, and then firmly against your seat.

The weights should be pushed back until they are just above your chest. Keep your palms pointing ahead. Reduce the weights slowly.

Breathe deeply as you lower the weights down and exhale as you lift.

Barbell Squat

Place a barbell on the upper part of your back. Do not place it on on your neck. Securely hold the bar using your hands that are twice shoulder width apart.

Your feet should be about the shoulder width apart and your toes must extend only slightly to the side by bending your knees in a manner.

Maintain the back of your body as straight as you can be allowed . While keeping your jaw forward, then twist your knees as you slowly allow your hips drop straight to the point at which your legs are in line with the floor. When you have reached the baseline position, you can push the weight back up to the initial position.

Be careful not to be hung on your shoulders or pivot to the side! A belt can be used to lessen the risk of lower back injuries. You can place your foot soles on a 1-inch square to work your quads.

You could also use an additional positioning to exercise on the quads of your internal muscles more.

Upright Barbell Row

Standing up straight, you can handle barbells with your hands approximately the width of your shoulders. Give the bar time to straighten out in front of you.

Maintain your wrists and body straight.

Then, push the bar upwards toward your button, while making sure it is close to your body.

Concentrate on pulling either using your traps or by the shoulder front depending on what want to accomplish the most.

Slowly lower until you reach the starting position. Do not cheat by turning either in the direction of forward or reverse. Make sure not to swing!

Front Dumbbell Raise

Maintain a dumbbell on each hand, palms facing each other in reverse. Your feet should be approximately shoulder width apart.

Maintain a slight twist in your elbows throughout the workout, making sure to ensure that you have straight arms, but not completely connected.

The weight should be lifted in your left side in before you, in a broad curve to the point at which it is just a little higher than the statue of the bear.

In a steady, controlled motion, lower the weight you are lifting the weight using your proper hand, so both arms are moving at the same time.

Be careful not to overdo it by using a swing or an incline in reverse! This lift should also be achievable using two dumbbells or the barbell.

Solid Leg Barbell

Set a barbell onto your shoulders. Keep your head straight until your back is straight. Then, bend your midriff and keep your legs locked, to you reach the point where your abdominal muscles are aligned with your floor.

Reverse slowly to the position you were in before. It is also possible by keeping your knees slightly bent.

One Leg Barbell Squat

Use a 12-18-inch box or a seat for this exercise The bigger your case is, the more challenging the task.

Put a barbell on your head near the neck's base. Use the barbell in two hands, using more than a the bear's width grip.

You should stand approximately 2 to 3 feet away from the container and rotate with the intention that the case is straight in front of you.

Begin by stepping one foot back. place your foot in the container. Make sure your opposite foot is level on the floor , and then put your toes forward.

Straighten your body. Keep your back straight and your chest straight throughout the exercise.

Keep your neck and head aligned to your middle, so that you're facing towards the future. Your shoulders must be completely finished on your front foot.

Keep your front foot flat with the floor place the hips forward (like you be sitting in a chair) and then twist the leg (of the leg in front) and slightly lean forward at the midriff.

Reduce your body slowly till your lower hip (of the front of your leg) is in line with the ground. In the event that you have difficulty dropping yourself to this level then lower yourself to your hip of the front leg has been bent 90 degrees.

The knee needs to be straight across your toe, and your hips should to be relaxed and your chest should to be finished in at the middle of your thigh.

Now, while driving with your chest and head and chest, lift your hips slightly to the side and upwards towards the roof.

You can then fix your leg. Reverse back to the starting position. Your shoulders should now to be completely finished on the in front.

Thrusts

Set a barbell to your back. Your chest should be lifted and gaze straight ahead. Place your right leg forward during a long walk.

Your foot should be at a sufficient distance from you to ensure that when you bend your knee correctly, your lower leg and your thigh form a perfect point.

Slowly twist your knees and lower your hips until your back knee is clear of the floor. Then, if you are able to do it quickly At this point, slowly straighten your legs and then raise your body up to a standing posture.

Complete a complete set, then switch legs and repeat, or swap legs after each repetition.

Be sure that your knee does not extend past your toes when you are when you are in a down position!

This could also be done by using dumbbells in both hands instead of the barbell.

Barbell Triceps Extension

Use a barbell by placing your hands that are a bit closer than the bear's width. Lay on a seat and then position your head to the highest point.

The bar should be raised at an appropriate distance.

The bar should be lowered in an upward movement behind your head until you reach the point at which your lower arms touch your Biceps.

Keep your arms in close proximity to your head. Return to your starting position.

This can also be done using the straight bar two dumbbells, positioned on a stand or standing, or with two dumbbells with your palms facing into.

The above-mentioned exercises can be done in an exercise studio or in your own home.

In the event that you join a recreation centre, they'll have many equipment that can work on specific regions in your body. The staff at the fitness center will be able to assist you in how to use the equipment.

If you know what tasks to perform, why don't we look at three or four examples of exercises.

Chapter 14: Protein And Muscle Growth

Protein is the most coveted nutrition for anyone who is a bodybuilder. Go to any store selling supplements or gym and you'll be subject to endless talks from experts on how crucial protein is to your progress as a bodybuilder. They will also tell you how much you must consume to maximize your muscle growth.

While protein is crucial in repairing muscles damaged by injury and to help rebuild muscles, it's unclear how much you'll need every day to ensure that you're providing sufficient protein to the body to replenish itself and get larger and more robust.

Our bodies are now stocked with diverse kinds of protein and all of them are involved in various tasks that include DNA replication, cell signaling and repair muscles and tissue and laying the foundation for other areas of your body, such as hair skin, nails, and even your hair. The protein that makes muscle requires an exact type of amino acid, referred to as the essential amino acid. These are not absorbed into the body and must be derived from food sources, which is why they are termed "essential" because the body requires them in order to remain alive.

When you eat food with protein, your body breaks down proteins into distinct amino acids that make the proteins needed by the body. In the building and repairing muscle tissue phase, your body utilizes all essential amino acids to make muscle protein and then connects a variety of proteins together in order to create new muscles.

If you don't consume enough proteins throughout your day you'll not have the amino acids that your body requires to repair muscle tissue which severely hinders the growth of any muscles that are lean. This is most likely the primary reason why nutritionists as well as personal trainers advocate high-protein diets. For non-bodybuilders, there is a minimum amount of protein on a every day basis for development and repair. However, when they engage in intense workouts (i.e. powerlifting) the need for amino acids is dramatically raised as their body is subject to a greater amount of stress and wear than an uninvolved person.

This is where we'll look into the "optimal" amount of protein intake to achieve gains in muscles This is among the most frequently-asked bodybuilding related questions.

How Much?

While this issue is frequently disputable, there's a wealth of research conducted in the field of science and nutrition for sports particularly in relation to the consumption of protein in absolute quantities and the timing of nutrient intake. The most recent meta-analyses conducted by professionals in the field, Alan Aragon, Brad Schoenfeld along with Eric Helms, sought to find the answer to this issue.

Research results from 49 separate studies involving 1,863 participants demonstrated that Schoenfeld's team discovered that the optimal intake of protein intake for athletic people (i.e the bodybuilders) can be ~1.6g/kg mass. 1

Following conducting the research, team made a conclusion that consuming protein in excess of 1.62 grams/kg/day led to the RET-induced decrease in FFM.

~0.74g/lb/day This is like the recommended 0.8g/lb bodyweight daily. While you're definitely not putting yourself at risk by eating more than 0.74-0.8g/lb/day of protein. However, that's unlikely to aid you in building muscles any more or speed up the process neither.

So, if you're a fan of foods that are protein-rich and feel they are more satisfying than carbs or fats and you're not worried about it, then that's great. But , it's probably better to put the calories you've saved towards oils (which are more filling and comforting) or carbohydrates (which will boost the performance of your body) instead.

Proteins of First Class and Second Class

The most important aspect of bodybuilding is tracking full forms of the protein (known in the first category) as well as incomplete proteins, also known as second class. They can be distinguished by the quantity of amino acids essential found in the food item.

A complete protein contains nine amino acids (Leucine, Isoleucine, Lysine, Methionine, Phenylamine, Threonine, Tryptophan, Valine and Histidine) necessary for our body. In this sense, any plant-based proteins you consume are complete protein.

Complete proteins are the basic muscles building blocks, also known in amino acids. They join to form conforming proteins, much like cars connecting to form an ultra-fast train, or perhaps letter of the alphabet that are put together to form words. For vegans, the most protein sources contain a substantial quantity of these nine essential amino acids However, not all of them contain sufficient amounts of all of them.

In particular, those who are vegan typically struggle to get a sufficient amount of Lysine since it becomes difficult when they don't consume enough legumes and soy-based products (such as soy meats tofu, tempeh , and soy milk) as well as beans (black pinto, garbanzo navy, fava etc.) and chickpeas (including falafel and hummus and so on.) and peas and peanuts or quinoa.

Depletion of Lysine could cause you'll be lacking in amino acids essential to your body. This could slow your progress in bodybuilding and could cause insufficient or slow recovery following training, depriving you of increase in muscle mass and increasing your risk of suffering an injury. Therefore, in order to prevent this, make sure you include at minimum two or three insufficient sources of protein into your mealsor take a assortment of colors and foods that you ought to already be doing. In the next chapter we'll give suggestions on how to cook vegan dishes, and also some suggestions for foods that will help you build the growth of your muscles.

How to prepare a vegan meal

If you are concerned to achieving the best results as a vegan , preparation of meals is the important factor. It is advantageous because you don't have to be concerned about your meat becoming rotten and it can also reduce your expenses, since meat and dairy aren't so affordable as fruits and starches. But, you need to be careful when the balance of a vegan diet in the same way as you would balance meals that contain meat. Here are some guidelines to help you simplify the process.

General tips on how to cook for meals.

Make sure you have a game plan in place prior to going out to buy food, as this will ensure that you're more likely stick to your plan once you've got one.

Write down everything you need to eat to get through the coming week (especially in the case of cooking with a variety of recipes) make a list of all the food items you need, then make sure you shop your groceries prior to.

Making batches of food will make cooking easier in the course of the week.

The most common ingredients are likely to be used again and if you are required to cook everything in one go it is a good idea to increase the quantity! The easiest items that you can cook up in batches are vegetables, brown rice as well as black bean spaghetti sweet potatoes, and tofu.

How to prepare vegan meals

There are two ways I go about my vegan food preparation. I usually use"ingredient preparation "ingredient prep" in warmer months, which is when I consume lots of smoothies and fruits as well as the "meal preparation" method during the winter months in which I eat more soups, curries, stews, and other meals which are hot. If my next week is likely to be full I may employ the prep method in which the weather is pleasant too.

Ideas for food preparation using vegan ingredients

Here's my usual vegan food preparation essentials. When I have these ingredients stored in the refrigerator, I can prepare simple meals at any time during the week. I don't prep every one of these meals every week and the ingredients could vary from week to week, but you should understand the basics. Wash and cut different vegetables bake some starch-based vegetables and cook protein-based dishes such as lentils and tofu, prepare some grains, in the event that you want.

Mince A big bowl of beets, carrots

Bake some spaghetti squash

Roast some the yams, butternut squash and sweet potatoes

Use dry ingredients to prepare containers to make the overnight Oats

Slice up carrot sticks, and celery

Chop up a portion of bell peppers in a bowl.

Prepare a lot of zucchini noodles

Bake some extra-firm tofu

Cook an array of edamame shells

Mix together a variety of grains such as rice or Quinoa

Take along some fruits on the go, such as dates or bananas for snacks.

Bowls and Containers

When your meals for the week been prepared, you'll require a method to preserve the food items. A majority of preppers use dishwasher and microwave-safe bowls for convenience of cleaning and use. Here are some guidelines to keep in mind when buying containers:

Different types of materials

It is vital to choose containers that aren't contaminated by BPA. If you're using the plastic container with BPA It could add chemicals that alter hormones to food items if you cook it for prolonged durations in a microwave or dishwasher.

Quantity and size of containers

Are you planning to prepare three meals each day of the week Are you seeking easy and easy lunches? Are you planning to make complete meals that include dishes and sides or maybe just a cup or breakfast cereal and banana in the day? Consider the number in terms of size, quantity, and types of meals you're familiar with and then purchase in accordance with the information you have gathered.

The number of compartments

Some containers consist of a single compartment and others contain at least three slots that allow you to organize food in a separate way. If you're planning to bring meals such as chili or stew or don't mind your food touching one another the one container might be enough. If you'd like to keep your grains, greens and proteins choose containers that are bento-style and is divided into slots.

While some containers are economical, starting at $10-15 for a 7-set container, you must make an effort to buy the highest quality that will be beneficial to you over the long run. Plastics that are made cheaply or recycled from take-out containers will fall apart quickly. While it may appear as a sensible option but it could cost you more in the long run when replacing the plastic.

Seal durability

Soupy or soupy meals that often "slosh" require containers that have sealed tightly or else you'll risk your food spilling out all over the interior of your bag or backpack.

You can eat what you like.

While I recommend preparing meals ahead of time but it's only effective in the event that you consume them throughout the week. So, make sure you're planning for meals you enjoy.

Green beans are easy to prepare since they can be prepared in large quantities. However, even if you're not keen on the taste of green beans it won't inspire you to think about staying with your diet.

It's an excellent idea to select foods that you enjoy and experiment with the combination and spices to ensure that you're never bored by their flavor.

Needs for nutrition in macros

Alongside the comfort of having food prepared to go straight out of the refrigerator food preparation can help you achieve targets for health and fitness.

Remember that your needs may also alter based on your sexuality and age. The needs of a 19-year-old girl may differ from that of the needs of a man who is 50 years old.

The process of preparing can be completed by anyone, however make sure that you plan out what macronutrients and calorie intake that your body needs.

Note your diet plans in a notebook

The key to success in the beginning of a vegan lifestyle isn't just in the food you consume, but as well having a clear understanding of the foods you consume. Human memory by itself isn't a reliable source of consciousness which is why making exact notes in a food journal is crucial in your progress.

This means that every bite of food you eat and every drink you consume throughout the day should be recorded. In the event that you don't, what you've learned will fade away from your mind as time passes It may be difficult initially however it will become more effortless over time.

For a newbie, if you're not equipped with the correct direction or the right information it is like lost in the storm with no compass and you're more susceptible to the harmful substances you consume and the stuff that is actually functioning.

Also, make sure you're prepared to eat correctly. If you're an avid snacker, you can avoid cravings throughout the day by using the fresh nuts you have in your kitchen and ripe bananas dried fruit, seeds. The convenience of having healthy food options in your pantry can make it easier and more convenient to snack on healthy food and stay healthy in the process.

Conclusion

I hope that this book is helpful in helping you gain greater understanding of the bodybuilding diet and offer specific advice on your nutritional goals and requirements.

It is the next stage to create your own menu plan or just try the meal plan that is provided from this guide. The duration of 4 weeks is enough to allow you to feel and observe the benefits of a regular diet.